CHICF
HAROLD WA

R0017238

D0290424

R00172 38321

REF

RA
412.5
.U6
W48

White, Ben B.

Falling arches

Cop. 1

DATE			

REF
RA
412.5
.U6
W48
Cop.1

Business/Science/Technology
Division

The Chicago Public Library

SEP 26 1978

Received_____

© THE BAKER & TAYLOR CO.

FALLING ARCHES

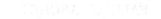

FALLING ARCHES

The Case Against Federal Intervention
in the Practice of Medicine

Ben B. White, M.D.

Exposition Press   *Hicksville, New York*

A collection of papers and letters
intended to help private practitioners
understand the mechanics of federal intervention
and how to defend against it with additional thoughts
on the socialization process in general.

FIRST EDITION

© 1977 by Ben B. White, M.D.

All rights reserved, including the right of reproduction in whole or in part, in any form or by any means, electronic or mechanical, including photocopying, recording, or by any information storage and retrieval system. No part of this book may be reproduced without permission in writing from the publisher. Inquiries should be addressed to Exposition Press, Inc., 900 South Oyster Bay Road, Hicksville, N.Y. 11801

ISBN 0-682-48871-2

Printed in the United States of America

BUSINESS/SCIENCE/TECHNOLOGY DIVISION
THE CHICAGO PUBLIC LIBRARY   SEP 2 6 1978

REF
RA
412.5
.U6
W48
Cop.1

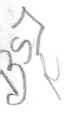

Contents

Preface

As a practitioner with thought patterns which are apparently on a different channel than those of my colleagues, it seemed necessary to commit those thoughts to paper in the manner of a mental cathartic to help relieve anxiety about the future of private practice and liberty.

The primary emphasis of this book is to analyze the forces which bring about socialized medicine and to offer corrective measures; but it is not possible to isolate this problem from the "socialization" process in general.

Not being a recognized "philosopher," nor even one trained in philosophy, nor a significant influence on medical matters, I had no alternative but to write a book to record what is perceived as "right." Law school courses were quite helpful in analyzing problems facing physicians.

A certain anxiety stems from a desire not to be simple and not to slip into the dark pit occupied by philosophers such as Plato, Rousseau, Robespierre, Marx, Hitler, etc., who may originally have been well motivated but who never achieved the understanding of individual man and his society necessary to enable them to come to grips with what I call the "vicious circle." Consequently, their efforts not only did not bring man to the peak of progress and tranquility but, on the contrary, fueled and fanned the basic fires which produce social conflict, the fires which fuel the vicious circle.

It would be of no benefit either to my mind or others to recycle those philosophies, but the present deteriorating world conditions and trends dictate overwhelmingly that further analysis of man's association is warranted.

Many of those men, during their lifetimes, realized the futility or rather the error of their ways, experienced and died with the frustration, which is so often the fruit of misguided zeal, without experiencing the satisfaction of a dilemma resolved. They were the nidus about which society's desires for tangible materialistic goals coagulated, desires which constantly seek a vehicle which will provide easy success, and thus they were nothing more than the personification of man's lack of understanding of himself. So mankind continues to suffer, by the millions, the consequences of its myopic cupidity.

Since the very early philosophers did not have the recorded experience of human association which modern man has, they should not be criticized too severely for being the nidus which catalyzed the coagulation of man's desires for the tangible into physical effort even though those efforts did result in such carnage. The same cannot be said for twentieth-century totalitarian leaders. Nevertheless, all their individual failures were the evidence of, the personification of society's failure as a whole, a society which continues with the same problems to produce the same type "leaders" with the same "visions" and the same ultimate end result. The vicious circle, in this late twentieth century, still goes on, and, as I pass by, I would like to try to throw at least one monkey wrench into this circle in an effort to stop it at a point which provides a mechanism for all societies to gain the peak of progress and tranquility, with the qualifications to hold it.

The prevention of socialized medicine would be a big monkey wrench.

Introduction

A politically influential and increasingly vocal group is demanding major changes in the "Health Care Delivery System." According to these critics, medical practitioners must be redistributed and the methods of delivery of service be restructured. It is almost certain that major changes will occur in the seventies.

A few criticisms may be valid, but the proposed overhaul is to be made without proper analysis of either the factors which have produced adverse socio-economic conditions or the probable detrimental effects of the proposed changes.

The medical profession has the ominous feeling that the changes will not be beneficial but in its confusion about the issues is unable to offer any better solution. The proposed new approaches such as National Health Insurance (NHI) will result eventually in all attention being given to economic issues and only lip service to the preservation of quality. Such misguided changes cannot accomplish the desired goals but, on the contrary, will aggravate existing conditions by fanning the fires of inflation, reducing the quality and availability of care, and producing a more chaotic situation in general, while depriving society of certain freedoms. The implementation of the proposed changes subjugates the entire matter of medical care to an untrained, politically motivated bureaucracy without providing the ballast necessary to control cost, utilization, and quality.

Part I
The Vicious Circle

1
Why History
Repeats Itself

With all his tangible material accomplishments, his vast knowledge of his environment, man has not yet discovered or developed an equation for successful human association, an equation which will provide permanently for his most desired goals of maximum prosperity and tranquility. Consequently and unwittingly, society continually conducts a haphazard search for a nebulous goal to satisfy its inherent drives, a nebulous goal which is called "Utopia." But man does not yet understand his inherent drives and therefore his search continues in a circle, a circle which causes untold suffering. He seeks Utopia unconsciously, dreamlike, without realizing that he is doing so and without understanding either what that goal is or the unfortunate consequences of his search, as that prize continues to elude him.

The present trend toward socialized medicine is but one manifestation of this historically recurrent process, a process which leads from freedom to slavery to freedom to slavery. The search is the result of society's failure in general, and government's failure specifically to fully understand the individual's inherent drives and to establish rules of association which cope with those drives so that man's most prized attainable goal, his freedom, can be retained. He must understand his Utopian drive and the impossibility of its success if he is to achieve and retain the "Ideal" government which can provide safety, comfort, and maximum possible liberty.

The force which causes man to exert his God-given physical and mental abilities, to labor, is his desire for the tangible safety and comfort for himself and those who depend on him. He recognizes that these tangibles are attained only by his labors and are proportional to his labors. He places great value on "absence of restraint" on his labors because experience dictates that he can best attain his goals in an atmosphere free of restraint. This "absence of restraint" is an intangible which he calls "freedom" or "liberty." But, unfortunately, a serious complicating factor in man's individual nature is that if he can attain the tangible security and comfort without labor and still have the intangible freedom, he will choose that pathway. Society therefore, is multiple individuals laboring, constantly seeking maximum security, maximum comfort, and complete freedom (no government) while harboring the basic desire that this be accomplished with no effort. If all can accomplish that with no effort, that is Utopia, the Impossible Dream.

But what is possible is a governing environment in which each is free to exert his inherent capacities, to labor, according to his desires so long as his efforts do not restrict or interfere with another's labors to achieve the same personal goals.

Early in his existence, man recognized that the similarities in needs and desires produced conflict, insecurity, as all labored for security and comfort. He recognized the necessity for "government" as an authority to restrict his freedom in order to settle equitably and peacefully any disputes which arose from his labors so that his needs could be attained in an atmosphere of safety. *He tolerates of necessity, not of basic desire,* this governmental restriction of his freedom and continually tries to subvert the governing authority for his own benefit, even at the expense of the labors and freedoms of others, if he can do so safely. So with government came "politics," the euphemistic label given to man's efforts to use his government to improve his own environment, to achieve his personal Utopia, at the expense of his fellow man's labors and freedom. Politics is the socially acceptable manifestation of man's subconscious rejection of government. He exerts pressure on his elected governing officials to obtain rules and regulations that peacefully, in the name of "Law" promote and protect his personal interests at the expense of the labors and freedom of others; i.e., through government, man tries to neutralize the purpose of government insofar as his own desires are concerned. Through politics, man continues his search for Utopia not consciously realizing that since Utopia is impossible, and security and comfort are proportional to labors, then any increase of security and comfort without increased effort on his part can only be at the expense of others' labors and freedom. He realizes only that with politics, the greater the number with similar goals, the greater the chances of his sucess. Unions are society's manifestation of that realization. Unions are ill omens for individual liberty. Man sacrifices certain of his intangible freedoms for the sake of the tangible "group gain." The group, through politics, works to subvert the government designed to protect the individual's liberty in order to obtain rules and regulations (Laws) which peacefully promote group interests at the expense of the remainder of society's labors and freedoms.

Here are the seeds of civil strife and destruction of the national purpose as stated in the Preamble to the Constitution. Through politics, the government is subverted. It begins to lose its purpose of protecting the freedom of the individual laboring for security and comfort. The individual's rights fade in significance as group politics produces new "Laws," "Labor Laws," "Civil Rights Laws," to govern the relationships of "large group vs. large group," i.e., "Labor vs. Management," "Race vs. Race," "Union vs. Union," and within each large group are individuals who have sacrificed certain freedoms "for the good of the group."

But not all are in unions, not all are in management. Eventually the isolated non-union, non-big group member of society finds his freedoms gone, sacrificed to big group interests without any benefit from that loss.

"Large group" against "large group" necessitates "new government," "bigger government," "more powerful government," because the judicial system designed to adjudicate "individual vs. individual" was not designed to and cannot cope with large group interests and problems. A burgeoning new government of "Labor Laws," "Civil Rights Laws," etc., develop as government becomes stronger, sacrificing individual liberty in order to maintain peace, to prevent civil war, as "large groups" seek group Utopia through politics until finally, if civil war does not occur beforehand, government is overcome by the largest and most powerful group which then becomes the governing authority, the dictatorship of the proletariat. And so it goes. If no one of exceptionally strong character comes forward—no Rousseau, no Robespierre, no Stalin or Hitler—to serve as the nidus about which the Utopian drive of the people can coagulate; if no "vehicle" to Utopia appears, then the people, under the same Utopian urge, through free elections, through the political process, over a few generations of "political winnowing," will produce one, a dictator equivalent to the worst who have arisen of their own ability and effort. Man continues on course in the vicious circle which leads to totalitarian destruction of his freedom and its results, deterioration of his environment, both of which are the reverse of his basic desire. As the totalitarian noose tightens, as freedom diminishes of necessity to maintain peace, and social stagnation and regression occur over generations, the desire for tangible security and comfort wane and the desire for the lost intangible freedom which is necessary for progress begins to grow with eventual revolution and a rededication to freedom— the circle goes on.

The origin of freedom's destruction is politics. Governing officials succumb to political pressure, which is large groups saying, "Give us greater security, greater comfort, and freedom with no additional effort on our part." But, to reiterate, greater security and comfort for one group without commensurate increase in effort by that group can be attained only by somehow acquiring or harnessing for themselves the labors and rights of others.

This is where the "Economy" becomes involved and how "Inflation" results from the vicious circle. The temporary alternative to relative "slavery" for the politically impotent individual-small group is to participate in the "Inflationary Spiral." The subject, man's labor, has, for convenience, been given monetary value which in turn is the basis for what is called "The Economy." The large groups demand greater security through higher wages without increase in labors. For political reasons, these demands are met and the cost passed on to the consumers whose labors are multiple and varied and who, in order not to suffer a loss (become slaves relatively), pass that loss on by raising their prices etc. But since the economy is one economy, and all are inextricably linked, the large groups soon feel the inflationary pinch of their initial demands and proceed to issue more demands, the result being the "Inflationary Spiral" as all follow by demanding more money without increased effort. This is the reason Socialists-Communists are so eager for "Unionism." Unionism is the key to destruction of the free-enterprise economy by inflation.

The only ways the inflationary spiral can be stopped are for the politically impotent groups to submit voluntarily to slavery, i.e. provide their services for a minimal fee with no increases due to inflation, or for government to control the wages of all. Of course, those with the greatest political influence will receive the most favorable treatment until a dictatorship is firmly established. Unfortunately, progress does not originate with the politically potent large group, but with the politically impotent individual-small group. In Socialism and Communism, progress, therefore, is exceedingly slow.

The end result of "Production Capacity" being converted from a primary goal of "First Rate Production" for the benefit of all, to one of insuring economic security for a few, is inflation for all and a form of slavery for many, if not all.

Political pressure is the energy source of the vicious circle, the Utopian circle. Politicians and social idealists succumb to this group pressure and destroy ideal government by piloting the search for Utopia.

The weapon which the politician uses to relieve the pressure on him is the art of compromise. Unfortunately for the advocate of individual liberty, of ideal government, the art of compromise is the art of graduated defeat. It is submission to the harness. And unfortunately for the advocate of liberty, there is no organized "large group" exerting political pressure for the intangible "liberty."

Some say that to defend our Constitution in its stated purpose to "secure the blessings of liberty to ourselves and our posterity," and to refuse compromise is to be a "Purist" or "Idealist" rather than a "Realist." To quote a favorite phrase, "We won't face up to and accept the world as it really is." The world is as it is, however, because of men who failed to analyze, to recognize and correct the weaknesses which destroy the ideal system. They refuse to stand by principle. They take the easy way out, the uninformed path of compromise. So the motion of the vicious circle continues, a motion fueled by the Utopian Dream, a motion piloted by politicians under political pressure, a motion navigated in its circular direction by compromise, a motion rolling again towards chaotic repression of individual liberty as it nears the dictatorial phase.

The motion can be stopped at the point of ideal government only because in this constitutional system, alone, lies both the mechanics and the freedom to do so.

The defense of ideal government is very logical. Ideal government provides for freedom as a matter of law. All that is needed is for the individual to recognize where his freedom is in jeopardy and assert the law. As citizens we have a moral duty to exert every effort to "secure the blessings of liberty to ourselves and our posterity." We must not allow the right to life, liberty, and the pursuit of happiness to be degraded by the political process and ground under the wheels of compromise. But only he whose freedom is threatened has the right and authority to defend it. *So each one must be vigilant.* By failure to recognize where your liberty is in danger and to defend it through established legal channels, your liberty is not taken from you—you forfeit it. That is how socialism creeps. The end result of the search for Utopia, i.e., socialism or totalitarianism, is not a self-propelled entity which can go forward of its own legal power. It is an ever-present evil that is sucked into the vacuum which is created when free men retreat by failure, usually through ignorance, to use the legal system, the government, designed for the purpose of preventing that event.

The history of government is the history of politics. Certainly that history does not invoke in one a strong desire to depend on politicians to preserve liberty. Politicians will not salvage your civil rights. They cannot. Your civil rights are their sustenance. Politicians must consume your civil rights in order to remain politicians. This is the reason for so few "conservative" politicians, true statesmen. The true statesman's goal is to preserve the intangible freedom, your civil rights. Statesmen do not exist at the expense of civil rights and therefore they have no "food" on which to survive. The true statesman has no organized "large group" driven by Utopian desires to exert political pressure on him. Politicians, on the other hand, thrive on such pressure and feel that they must respond through their only available weapon, compromise—and the motion continues . . .

We must act individually. Each of us must decide what his individual policies will be. Will ignorance, fear, and apathy prevail or will informed effort preserve your freedom? Will you be true to principle, or will you be your own Judas? Will you say, "Conscience, Conscience, where art thou?" and be a party to untold misery for future generations; or will you stand fast and defend the principles of individual freedom? Are we to rationalize ourselves into retreat before the compromise machine or do we resist with "law" in a war where differences in numbers need not be the determining factor in victory but victory, rather, is determined solely by the ability and willingness to use your weapon.

We have an unbeatable weapon with which to defend against encroachment on our freedom, but each one must use it. Each one must have an understanding of that weapon if he is to be successful. Therein lies our greatest weakness. You must learn something of the law which governs our associations. Then you can successfully defend your freedom with a spirit of compassion towards your fellowman who would take it, the same spirit as One who died on the Cross saying, "Forgive them, Father, for they know not what they do."

St. Mark said, "What shall it profit a man if he gain the whole world and lose his soul?"

What shall it profit a society if it gain maximum security but forfeit its freedom?

Part II
Socialized Medicine: Cause and Prevention

2
Sequence of Events—
The Why of Federal Control

For physicians, the basic knowledge they must have, must thoroughly understand, so that it can be applied in all their office-hospital relationships is this:

Under the Constitution, the Thirteenth Amendment, you are an "independent contractor." This is the legal terminology for "freedom" or "liberty." The designation "M.D." does not change that status; it does not change your relationship to the civil statutes which govern this nation. Your civil rights are unchanged. You have no greater authority over any others nor do any others have any greater authority over you. You have assumed, by virtue of your license, the single additional legal duty of rendering medical care and advice with reasonable care and skill when requested to do so and you agree to do so.

Third-party economic and political interests must have the use of your license for the success of their political-economic (Utopian) purposes. They will try any manner of subversion of your civil rights to obtain use of that license.

These forces of evil must accomplish two goals to be victorious in their efforts. They must (1) gain control of the physician's income, and (2) gain control of the physician's license.

Such control is socialized medicine.

There are many mechanisms of "why" they must control the doctors and "how" it is intended to be accomplished. These are dealt with in greater detail elsewhere. Suffice it to say that physician income is to be controlled at the office level through physician ignorance of assignment law while loss of control over his license is to occur at the hopsital level through so-called "Utilization Review" and "Delineation of Privileges," both to be accomplished through the agency of the JCAH (Joint Commission on Accreditation of Hospitals) as "Conditions for Accreditation."

Success on their part will be through subversion of civil rights, through physician forfeit, which is no legal violation.

So you *must* understand your civil rights in relationship to third parties both in your office and your hospital associations if you are to preserve those civil rights, your freedom, and thereby preserve your ability to abide by Section VI of the AMA Code of Ethics.

In order for federal control of medical care to occur, government must have a political "why" it must control physicians and hospitals and a legal "how" to obtain that control.

When pressures build in a free society so as to encourage federal intervention, those pressures are the tangible issues of inflation of the service concerned (rising costs) and lack of availability of the service concerned.

If those pressures build so as to provide a favorable political foundation for federal intervention, i.e., government doing for the people without public dissent and even with public approval, those pressures are but the result of failure of government to provide a proper legislative and judicial environment in which people can do for themselves. People doing for themselves is a free society, the free enterprise system. When government intervenes with its rules and regulations, its additional restrictions, it can do no more than the people would have done for themselves under the proper governing atmosphere and without loss of liberty.

In other words, the necessity for federal intervention is the result of original federal negligence. And what hope is there for a falling rock to reverse its course?

Certainly the American public has cause for concern about the rising cost of medical care and its lack of avaliability to large segments of the population except as wards of the government.

Those who study the problem however seem to do so only with the purpose of finding a politically acceptable way to pay for the problem. More attention must be given to the socio-economic forces which have caused the problem and have thereby provided the emotional-political foundation for governmental intervention. Only by correcting the cause will a lasting solution be found and the national purpose, as so well stated in the Preamble of the Constitution, be served.

Most of those who are concerned with the health care crisis seem to regard it as of recent virgin birth rather than the expected product of a forty-year gestation of certain socio-economic events. The following is an effort to examine those events, their consequences, and the role of governmental negligence in their development, the latter being a relatively untouched subject even though it is the primary cause of the problem.

To begin with, consider certain basic points about the concept of "insurance." The insurance industry, which is supposed to operate according to state laws, is, from a practical viewpoint, the implementation of free-enterprise economic theory for preventing socio-economic conditions that would so jeopardize the economic independence of middle- and low-income people that governmental intervention would be necessary for their economic salvation. The "jeopardy" or crisis which is the threat to that economic independence is "inflation" and its spin-off, "lack of availability of the service concerned" to those who need it. Insurance is the free-enterprise equivalent of the socialist concept "from each according to his ability, to each according to his need." Like its socialist counterpart, it is designed to provide all citizens with economic access to needed facilities and services, but on a voluntary non-regimented basis. *It must be recognized that the economic integrity of any insurance plan (including those of government) is dependent on the idea that individuals pool their resources to protect themselves at minimal expense against crippling financial loss as the result of real events the occurrences of which are not within the power of the insured. Any insurance plan will be economically sound only if the premiums are used to pay the expenses of statistically measurable events. Only when this definition and intent of insurance is abused will crisis in the form of inflation occur.* The duty to see that the insurance industry is operated according to definition and economic intent lies with government. *Failure to understand or recognize this truth forms not only a socio-economic foundation favorable for governmental intervention but also serves as the reason government finds it necessary to insert Utilization Review, Recertification, and PSRO (Professional Standards Review Organization) in its program.*

What is the abuse which produces this crisis called inflation? What is this abuse which is the father of Utilization Review, Recertification, and PSRO *whose very presence indicates lack of understanding of why they are needed?* What is the reason the free enterprise system is not accomplishing the purposes of Utilization Review, Recertification, and PSRO for the private insurance industry? In a word, the abuse is "over-utilization." What then is over-utilization? From a practical viewpoint, *over-utilization is the use of facilities for uninsurable purposes* (i.e., not medically necessary). Why and how does it come about?

Prior to World War II, before health insurance was even an embryo and later while health insurance was in its infancy, medical care was primarily concerned with diagnosis and treatment of symptomatic illness. It consisted of the care of illness, surgery, and trauma. This was and still is the basis of medical school training and the practice of medicine. Hospitals are our system's progressive means of mating patient needs with scientific progress. The concept of health insurance developed as a free enterprise economic adaptation to this improved but more expensive health care. But what has happened? Why a crisis? Why over-utilization?

With post-World War II advances in medical science's decreasing the frequency and severity of acute illnesses and thereby increasing longevity, with advances in communications producing a public with a greater understanding and awareness of disease, and with improved transportation providing easier access to medical facilities, medical practice has undergone considerable change. It is now composed of three categories.

INSURABLE:

I. Acute or short-term illness, surgery and trauma
   A. *Requiring hospital care*
   B. *Requiring out-patient care*

INSURABLE:

II. Chronic or long-term illness including so-called catastrophic illness
   A. *Requiring hospital care*
   B. *Requiring nursing-home care*
   C. *Requiring only home care*

UNINSURABLE:

III. Preventive medicine
   A. *Public Health medicine*
   B. *Early Detection Procedures (EDP) and Diagnostic Procedures*

The Public Health category is not pertinent to the crisis because its primary function is prevention of disease in the population-at-large rather than detection and treatment in individuals. Its functions do not involve the individual citizen's financial resources to any significant degree, are not a threat to his financial security, and are not a significant factor in over-utilization of medical facilities.

Early Detection Procedures, however, are a significant cause of over-utilization. EDP refers to studies which are done in an effort to detect disease before it becomes symptomatic. These studies, usually negative, are *initiated* by a public made "disease-conscious" by the joint educational efforts of the communications media and organized medicine, i.e., by progress.

Diagnostic Procedures are those studies requested by a physician in the exercise of his training and judgment (license). Many of these will be negative due to the nature of man's inherent inadequacies, i.e., his lack of X-ray and microscopic visual ability.

When the health insurance concept was implemented during the 1930s, it was designed primarily for Category I problems. Since WW II, the insurance concept has been *unjustly* strained by the added burdens of Categories II and III. The concept is faltering. This does not mean that the concept is invalid, but only that it is not being properly implemented; it is being abused.

Category I (Acute illness, surgery, trauma) is an insurable entity because these are real events produced by accidents or acts of God.

Category II (Chronic Illness) also is an insurable entity, but many of this Category II B and II C do not require hospital facilities. Hospital occupancy by II B and II C is over-utilization.

But Category III B is *not* an insurable entity because it represents expenditures limited only by the medically uneducated patients' desire to initiate a search for insurable entities (disease), so long as someone else pays the cost of that search. And in all three categories must be included the over-utilization caused by the physician's educated diagnostic efforts. *The economic system, i.e., the insurance industry, has not adapted to this aspect of health care because the fact that the search for illness is not an insurable entity has not been recognized.* Category III B, this non-insurable entity, funded by insurance premiums, is the primary destructive force in the economics of health care. It is this force which is destroying the free enterprise concept of health insurance by inflation and therby providing a political foundation for Federal intervention, i.e. a "crisis."

Category III is sustained and nourished by four factors which have an inflationary effect on free enterprise medical economics, i.e., four factors which promote over-utilization.

One factor which should be corrected by the legislature or judicial system by legal definition is the ability of an insured to collect more than the insured loss by owning multiple policies. One should be free to buy as many policies as he desires, but by the legal definition of insurance be allowed to be reimbursed only to the extent of his economic loss. The insurance industry ineptly tries to perform this government function by its duplicate coverage clauses.

A second factor is the ability to collect insurance monies without having incurred a loss—an event completely incompatible with the insurance concept but yet fostered by negligent government. This is the factor which forces many physicians to take assignments. Most people, in the emotional atmosphere of paying for health care services, forget that the *purpose* of *health insurance* is to *insure* payment of the doctor bill and hospital bill. Insurance contracts try to accomplish that purpose by having "Proof of Loss" contingency in the contract. This provides that where the doctor does not take assignment, the patient must furnish "Proof of Loss," not proof of illness, but proof of financial loss as a result of that illness. At present, however, the insurance industry, in violation of its Charters, accepts a doctor's bill as "Proof of Loss" when in reality it is only notice of debt. The company pays the patient a certain sum based on the bill serving as "Proof of Loss" and at this point the purpose of the contract i.e., payment of the doctor bill can be easily defeated by the patient.

This basic illegality is the reason so many physicians must resort to assignment in order to be paid for their services; and if they are not informed of the law of assignment become easy prey for third-party economic controls. Physicians can circumvent the above illegality by refusing to furnish the patient with diagnosis and treatment until the bill is paid at which point it can be marked "Paid" and then becomes legal "Proof of Loss." A promissory note is sufficient to allow a bill to be marked "Paid."

A third, and probably the most inflationary factor, is the over-utilization caused by the inherent willingness of one to advance or protect his own interests at any expense (check-ups etc., i.e., a search for illness) so long as the expense is someone else's. (All a result of the Utopian drive.)

A fourth factor is the over-utilization inherent in a physician's educated efforts to diagnose illness.

If home fire insurance were handled today as health insurance is, there would be a shortage of contractors, architects, and builders. The average home would cost $100,000 and as a result many would be without homes. This of course would set the stage for federal intervention and Homecare.

These four factors are destroying the free enterprise method of providing all citizens with the ability (insurance) to pay for real illness. These factors have caused such an increase of expenditures by over-utilization that the resulting inflation is forcing large numbers of those *for whom the concept of insurance was designed* out of the private health care system into the Federal lap while conditioning this same unwitting and large group to support federal control as the only means of obtaining medical care at reasonable prices.

These factors have brought doctor against doctor, doctor against government, doctor against hospital, doctor against insurance company, and even doctor against patient because of "over-utilization," Utilization Review Committees, "Recertification," "Peer Review," Drug Formularies, Usual, Reasonable, and Customary, Fee Schedules, Relative Value Scales, PSRO, etc. If these wrongs were corrected, there would be no inflated economic foundation on which political leverage could be obtained to promote such economically disastrous compensatory programs as Medicare and Medicaid.

The answer to the problem of course is to prevent hospital occupancy by Category II B, II C and III B, leaving these facilities only for Category I and II A.

Some of this would be resolved if the insurance industry would offer coverage for Category I and II as separate plans. Much would still depend however on successfully dealing with over-utilization caused by III B.

It is proposed that the dilemma of III B be solved by:

1. Establishing a mechanism under the law which would enforce the insurance *intent* by definition that no profiting be allowed on insurance; and by

2. Causing the insurance industry *not* to be responsible, again by definition, for laboratory, radiological and other expenses

where no pathological, radiological or clinical diagnosis is established. *This is what insurance is all about.*

It cannot be denied that EDP are important. It is not desired that preventive medicine be abolished. The nature of the human being is, however, that he must have some personal motivation to spend his money. The low incidence of disease is not adequate motivation for expenditure of one's money for EDP.

A most effective motivation would be to allow a large percentage or all of such cost, to be deducted from income tax due. This would encourage a much larger segment of the population to have out-patient check-ups, and reserve hospital facilities for significant illness.

This approach would end the over-utilization stress on hospital facilities by promoting out-patient diagnostic studies. It would terminate spiraling hospital costs caused by severe over-utilization. It would nullify the need for Utilization Review, and PSRO by third parties. It would retain the freedom of all citizens, and preserve a high quality of medical care.

Medicare and Medicaid, as compensatory answers to basic economic wrongs but yet implemented in the same manner, have greatly magnified the problem. National Health Insurance Plans or any other plans not based on an understanding of the cause of the "crisis" will exaggerate the problem in catastrophic proportions.

Medicare and Medicaid could be eliminated and national health plans prevented *by public choice* by abolishing the political reason for their existence. This means the "Insurance" concept must be implemented according to its definition and intent. If this should happen, free enterprise would again be able to offer all a better insurance program than government without loss of basic freedom and with progressive improvement of care.

It must always be remembered that "when pressures build in a free society so as to force federal intervention, or to encourage it without dissent from the public, these pressures are but a reflection of failure of government to perform its primary duty of providing a legislative and judicial atmosphere in which people would automatically do for themselves. People doing for themselves is the free enterprise system. When government intercedes to do for people, it can do no more than that which the people would have done for themselves automatically, more efficiently, and without loss of basic freedom under a proper judicial and legislative environment."

Contrary to a Texas lieutenant-governor's opinion that "twentieth-century medicine is a technology shackled by a nineteenth-century delivery system," the truth of the matter is that twentieth-century medicine is shackled in its efforts to deliver quality medical care by sixteenth-century government, government that refuses to combine twentieth-century intelligence with reasonable analysis, government that refuses to abide by its own law, government that uses emotion as a primary weapon to attack a complex problem, government that is to say the least, archaic if not juvenile in its approach to this modern-day problem.

3
Psychological Warfare

In the war to socialize medicine, as in other wars, propaganda or psychological warfare is one of the enemy's weapons. The public has been conditioned for Federal control by the phrase "rising costs of medical care." This is an economic reality which however is the result of the previously mentioned but *unpublicised failure of government to perform properly in the field of insurance,* a failure which has led to massive over-utilization of health care personnel and facilities with resulting massive pouring in of third party funds which in turn is the prerequisite for inflation of the health care economy. Government does not recognize this relationship and therefore tries only to control those factors which are responsible for cost, i.e., doctors and hospitals, while exerting no effort of its own to control utilization which determines third party expense. By lumping these two problems together under "rising costs," the public and providers are conditioned for control of providers. The providers also are so confused about their role in health care economics that their uncertainty about the nature of events diminishes their will to resist federal encroachment.

Everyone then is more or less convinced that federal control (National Health Insurance or some other form of socialized medicine) will solve the problem of "rising costs." Under NHI or whatever form of socialized medicine, the true problem of over-utilization, i.e., rising third party expenses, will continue unabated but no longer publicized because it is no longer a public concern, no longer a strong political issue, because the public no longer pays. As a growing government problem, it will

necessitate more and more controls over the few politically impotent providers of care with greater loss of liberty and poorer
quality of care as government continues an economic squeeze
on the providers trying to make them do what they can't do,
which is to keep third-party expenses down in a manner of
squeezing a fork harder and harder to make it a better utensil
with which to eat soup. Finally the fork is so bent, so abused, it
no longer can do what it was designed to do—and so it is with
doctors and hospitals under Socialized Medicine.

Another aspect of the psychological warfare is "Medical Care
as a Right," and again the providers are to bite the dust. A right
is the freedom to exercise God-given physical and mental capabilities to promote and protect one's interests. Individual responsibility is the exercise of those capabilities, the exercise of those
rights. A privilege, on the other hand, is the exercise of one's
rights jointly with others.

Government is the authority which provides the restraints
necessary to allow for the exercise of rights and privileges in a
safe and peaceful atmosphere, to progress. When a governing
atmosphere exists in which one's efforts, one's services, are another's rights, then slavery exists for the provider of those
services. Thus, regardless of what the propagandists say, medical
care cannot be a right unless physicians are slaves.

4

Utilization Review—
Points of Conflict
and Confusion

In 1965, in anticipation of Medicare, the AMA copyrighted a book entitled, *Utilization Review* (UR) which expresses the AMA's philosophy on this subject. The five-page introduction demonstrates inability to understand the purpose of Section VI of the AMA Code of Ethics, an inability to separate legitimate physician interest and responsibility from third-party interest and responsibility, an inability to separate responsibility for quality control from responsibility for cost control. This hang-up is the cause of present friction between physicians, hospitals, and government and is the father of those threats to professional freedom known as UR and PSRO.

The AMA, thus early in the game, demonstrated inability to recognize certain issues as matters not of ethics and therefore not within the realm of physician responsibility but rather as matters of *economics* and therefore in the realm of third-party economic responsibility. These problems were to be greatly magnified when government, as another and larger *economic* interest, appeared on the health care scene. The AMA either caused or allowed third-party economic responsibility to be shifted to the shoulders of physicians in the form of those threats to physician freedom and quality care, euphemistically known as UR and PSRO.

In its opening paragraph, the UR manual properly recognizes physicians as the sole responsible party for quality. In the next paragraph, however, it very smoothly executes Section VI of the Code of Ethics with the statement, "In recent years, however, a *new dimension* has been added to *appraisal of health care*—[emphasis added] appraisal of whether the use of hospital facilities was appropriate." In its confusion, the AMA identified the "new dimension" in health care as "appraisal of whether the use of hospital facilities was appropriate" rather than properly identifying the "new dimension" as the "third-party insurance industry economic interest in health care." By so mis-identifying, the AMA erroneously places certain responsibilities on physicians as matters of ethics rather than on the insurance industry as matters of economic policing.

By quoting figures on and calling the problem "rising hospital occupancy" rather than "rising third-party expenditures," the AMA deluded itself into believing that physicians have an ethical duty to police third-party expenditures under the cover of that euphemistic phrase, "Was this hospitalization appropriate?" i.e., "Was it medically necessary?" (so-called Utilization Review).

Physicians have the duty only of appraising or policing quality of care. They do not have the duty of policing the economic issue of "Who will pay for the care?" by policing the issue of *where* the care will be received. Physicians do not have the authority to police "where." They only recommend "where." The final authority for "where" is an inherent constitutional right of the patient, a decision based on consideration of the doctor's recommendation plus desire for care *balanced* (Utilization Curtailment) by the patient's financial ability. Ballast for desire for service, i.e., Utilization Curtailment, is and always must be economic in nature. It must be exercised either by the recipient of services in consideration of his personal economic status or by the third-party who, through that economic instrument known as an insurance policy, has assumed the patient's financial responsibility. Physicians, as providers of the requested service concerned, cannot properly restrict the use of that requested service anymore logically or effectively than a grocer can restrict the visits and expenditures of his customers. Such ballast, such curtailment, must come from the side of the recipient of services.

In other words, to be effective, utilization curtailment must be front-sided. Factors curtailing utilization must be applied before the decision of where the service will be provided is made and before the requested service is provided rather than as back-sided retrospective policing after the decision of where is made and the service begun. One uses certain measures to judge whether a lawn needs watering before the sprinkler is activated, not an hour or so after the sprinkler is on because the factors used to judge need have been altered. Utilization curtailment is a patient-third-party duty. To be effective, it must be in the form of front-side economic restrictions inherent in the nature of the third-party plan offered rather than back-sided or retrospective policing efforts by providers of care.

Utilization Curtailment, being a policing chore, is politically undesirable. The third-party dilemma was how to switch this politically undesirable responsibility, i.e. the job of saying "no" to those who desire the service but don't need it, and which the patient transferred to the carrier via his policy, from the carrier on to the physician.

With the quoted "new dimension" statement, the AMA volunteered its members to solve the third party dilemma. It volunteered physicians to be the ones to say "no." With that statement, the AMA allowed the "new dimension," the third-party insurance industry, to use physicians to interject economizing issues into the doctor-patient relationship in direct violation of Section VI of the Code of Ethics.

The integrity of Section VI must be maintained. Section VI is the recognition that recipients of care, of course, have an interest in cost of medical care. It is a recognition that, through the physician, cost and quality become related. It is a recognition that cost is a threat to quality if it is allowed to have full priority over quality. It is a recognition that the voluntary assumption by third parties of the patient's economic interest in health care does not place on them the duty to protect quality. It is a recognition, therefore, that since physicians are the point at which cost and quality meet and are balanced, and since physicians are solely responsible for quality, they must not allow themselves to be subjugated to rules and regulations controlling third-party expenditure lest physicians become the means, the agent through which economizing efforts are reflected as economizing or poor quality care. Physicians therefore must not be subjugated to rules and regulations concerning Utilization Review.

With UR, however, and much to the joy of the third-party concerned, physicians voluntarily assumed the politically undesirable task of policing third party expenditures according to third-party rules and regulations. By so doing, they voluntarily placed themselves in the double jeopardy position of not only relieving third parties of the responsibility for rising cost of medical care but also of assuming responsibility for any deterioration of quality which may come about as the result of third-party economizing efforts. Third parties, specifically Medicare, with physicians' help thus succeeded in the assassination of Section VI. This assassination was the first step on the long road to economizing second rate health care, the long road to socialized medicine. The trend can still be reversed; Section VI can still be revived but only by physicians.

The real problem is that physicians who are unable to analyze and cope with UR will be unable to analyze and cope with future questions such as, "Was the use of this drug or that procedure appropriate?" Those questions will be decided according to third-party rules. Those physicians will be totally socialized physicians, physicians whose licenses are manipulated and prostituted by bureaucrats for political gain, physicians who no longer have any control over the quality of care they dispense, physicians who have forfeited their civil rights, physicians who have lost their freedom.

In summary, many physicians, due to the AMA's misguidance, confuse the economic function of Utilization Curtailment with the ethical duty of peer review and remain convinced that Utilization Curtailment not only should be done by physicians but that the law requires this. They are in grievous error on both accounts, error which, by forfeit, forms the foundation for socialized medicine.

5
Physician Civil Rights and Third Parties

The greatest obstacle in the physician's battle to prevent socialization is his inability to understand what the socialization process is. He knows it is government control. But what is government control?

Control means authority. The gain by one party of authority over another means the loss of the latter's legal rights, i.e., his civil rights. Socialized medicine means that government gained authority over *individual* physicians that it did not have; i.e., *individual* physicians lost certain legal rights or civil rights which were transferred to government as authority over those *individual* physicians. Socialized medicine is the end result, therefore, of loss of *individual* physician civil rights. Since civil rights are constitutionally guaranteed, there is no way socialized medicine can occur by force of legislation. Socialized medicine, then, is the end result of loss of the civil rights of private practitioners *by forfeit. There is no illegality in forfeiture.* The problem, then, is getting physicians, individually, to understand where this forfeit is occurring so that they can understand how to stop this process at the office and hospital staff level at no expense to themselves.

There are certain very *basic* concepts which physicians, individually, must understand if the socialization process is to be halted.

The basics are as follows:

The ability to alter the environment in order to enhance his personal comfort and security is a manifestation of that capacity called "intelligence" which distinguishes man from other animals. The continual improvement of the environment is called "progress." Homo sapiens has learned through the ages that his mind harbors an intangible entity called "free will." He guards this free will very jealously because it is through this that he provides for his comfort and security. He has learned that the fewer the restrictions on his free will, the greater his ability to progress. He has learned, therefore, to prize absence of restraint on his free will. This absence of restraint he calls "freedom" or "liberty," and he naturally abhors restrictions, which he calls "imprisonment" or "slavery." The exercise of his free will to obtain comfort and security is called the exercise of "individual responsibility." Man has long sought the government which exerts the minimal restraint necessary to allow maximum progress in his society. This government was finally realized with the United States Constitution, primarily in the Thirteenth Amendment's prohibition of involuntary servitude. This amendment, being a generalization, was transferred to practical rules of association as those two basic rules of contract law which provide that:

RULE I:

Two parties are free to contract as they see fit so long as that contract does not interfere with the rights of others, does not violate criminal statutes, and does not violate public policy. This rule provides the atmosphere of minimal restraint which allows maximum progress through the relatively free exercise of Individual Responsibility.

RULE II:

No two parties can contract for the services of a third party and have force of law enforce performance by that third party. This rule prohibits coercion, or involuntary servitude, or slavery.

To illustrate these two rules:

A says to B, "I will pay you $10 if you mow my lawn." B agrees. The law then requires A to pay B the $10 if B mows the lawn or requires B to mow the lawn if A pays him the $10. This is freedom of contract and encourages association for mutual benefit or progress. (Rule I)

If A says to B, "I will pay you $10 *if* "C" mows my lawn." The law will not force C to mow the lawn (Rule II). But if C is ignorant of his basic Thirteenth Amendment civil right, and B can convince C that he has a legal or ethical duty to mow the lawn, then no law has been violated and there has been no involuntary servitude. C just forfeited his civil right through ignorance. THIS IS WHERE PHYSICIANS ARE TODAY!

The Medicare program is the prime example of the ABC illustration. As written, the "Medicare Law" does not violate any physician civil rights. As an insurance program, it is a manifestation of Rule I, the freedom of contract. It does not violate Rule II, the prohibition of involuntary servitude. It was very carefully written with careful and inconspicuous use of the word "If" so as to avoid that pitfall, while placing the unwitting physician in the position of the party C in the ABC illustration. Through ignorance, physicians continue to "mow the lawn" not knowing that their effort is not "required."

Section 1801 (a) of Public Law 89-97, the Medicare Law, states that "nothing in this Title shall be construed to AUTHORIZE [emphasis added] . . . any supervision or control over the practice of medicine. . . ." Medicare, as an insurance program, regardless of who the carrier is, is a contractual relationship (Rule I) between government, hospitals, patients, and intermediaries. No physician is a party to this Medicare contractual relationship. Section 1801 is a recognition of that fact and of Rule II in the basic law of contract under the Thirteenth Amendment. This means that nothing in the law can legally interfere with the physician's legal right, his civil right, to exercise his license as he and his patient see fit. Since that section is part of the law, it is also law. Any provisions later in the law that do interfere with this freedom to practice would be unlawful. The fact is, however, that no subsequent provisions in PL 89-97 even attempt, with force of law, to so interfere except Section 1842 (b) (3) (ii) to be touched on later. The problem is that physicians, because of negligent high level legal advice, think that PL 89-97 does require of them certain things such as Utilization

Review and Recertification. *The Medicare Law does not now and never has required those things of physicians.*

To illustrate:—Section 1814 (a) is an outstanding example of the ABC illustration. It makes no provision for mandatory Utilization Review and Recertification. That would violate Section 1801. It merely states that the hospital, as a party to the Medicare contract, will be paid only *"if"* a physician does Utilization Review and Recertification. It leaves it to the wiles of the administrator acting through the ignorance of the staff to accomplish that. It is an attempt to place the physician in the position of being a bad guy in that if he doesn't do something, the poor Medicare patient will lose his benefit. At law, this is not true. If it were true, then physicians could void the entire Medicare program, which they claim not to like, just by refusing to do Utilization Review and Recertification. The legal fact is that under the doctrines of either Promissory Estoppel or Substitute Performance, the hospital bill of a Medicare patient must be paid regardless of whether physicians, who are no party to the Medicare program, do Utilization Review and Recertification or not. The problem is that only the hospital or patient can sue HEW (Health Education and Welfare) on this question because only they would be the injured party through breach of contract. Physicians can, however, *at no cost,* solve the entire Utilization Review and Recertification problem just by exercising their constitutional right not to do it and thereby force the issue to court as "Hospital vs. HEW," a suit which the hospital cannot possibly lose since HEW itself has recognized its contractual duty by the statement that "no party or parties except Department of HEW can be held responsible for a Medicare patient's hospital bill."

Wilbur Cohen's best friends are those physicians who do to one another that which he knows he can't legally do, and that is to penalize one another for failure to do that which they have no duty to do. Hospitals and physicians must learn that their proper course of action is against HEW. Physicians have no duty to *any* third party carrier unless they take assignment for personal services and then they owe to that third party *no more* than diagnosis and medical description of services rendered.

6

The Law of the Land—
What Is It?

The statement "It is the law of the land" is seen frequently in various medical publications and often heard from medical leaders. It is made primarily in reference to Utilization Review, Recertification, and PSRO and is written or spoken with a defeatist attitude which indicates that the speaker or writer has thrown in the towel, exhausted his capacity to resist federal control of his practice, and will now respond as a robot to federal dictates. Since acceptance of the connotation of that statement is equivalent to total surrender, that phrase is in dire need of critical analysis.

First and foremost, the "law of the land" is not necessarily determined by Congress. It is often determined by the judicial system. It is to this division of government, the courts, that many questions should be brought in order to determine just what is the law of the land insofar as certain portions of the Medicare program are concerned. It is very important *how* these issues reach the courts.

No program passed by Congress and signed by the President is the law of the land until any question raised by that law, and involving the civil rights of any citizen, is made an issue by that citizen who, by the appropriate act, forces that issue into the courts for their determination of just what the law of the land is by interpreting the issue raised in the light of existing statute and ultimately the Constitution. Some issues become law through failure of the concerned party to cause the issue to become a court case. By forfeit then, the opposite of true law is implemented, as the citizen whose right is at stake fails to use the legal system designed to preserve that right. He forfeits his civil right, and that is how Socialism, *the opposite of true law, creeps forward.*

The doctor's civil right is the law of the land but he must claim it in order to make it so. The greatest single obstacle which we face is the failure of physicians to understand that socialized medicine is the end result of sacrifice without a fight of physician civil rights. Those rights cannot be lost if defended. Physicians simply do not understand where this forfeit is occurring. So where is it occurring? What is the doctor's civil right; what *is* the law of the land insofar as Utilization Review, Recertification, and PSRO are concerned?

The speakers and writers previously mentioned assume that Utilization Review, Recertification, and PSRO are "required" of physicians by PL 89-97. This is the most basic falsehood which is the foundation for all our problems with federal intervention. PL 89-97, the Medicare program, is by definition and title, an "Insurance Program" for the elderly. As such, it is a contractual relationship between government, intermediaries, hospitals, and a group of individuals age sixty-five years or over. The physician is not a party to that relationship. He pays no premiums; he signed no forms. He is no more a party to that relationship than to private health insurance relationships which non-medicare patients have.

The most basic "law of the land" is:

1. Two or more parties are free to contract as they see fit.
2. No two parties can contract for the services of a third party.

The parties to the Medicare program are free to do as they desire (1) but they cannot legally involve the physician in any manner against his will (2) except by his forfeit.

Thus, there is not, and cannot be any "requirement" of the physician by Medicare. Medicare "requires" the hospital, a party to that relationship, to have Utilization Review and Recertification. At law, that "requirement" is unenforceable, null and void. Medicare "requests" physicians to do it. Physicians do not have to do Utilization Review, Recertification, and PSRO. Whether they do it or not, the Medicare patient's hospital bill must be paid according to his contractual right.

And that, my fellow physicians, *is* the law of the land, but only physicians by claiming their right to protection under item 2 above, a corollary of the Thirteenth Amendment, can have that law, the real law of the land, implemented.

7

Basic Requirements
for Federal Control

THE "HOW" OF FEDERAL CONTROL

As man is entrapped in eternal conflict, war between the forces of freedom and those of slavery, the physician, in his area of involvement, must fight for his freedom on two fronts, the hospital and the office. On each front, several separate battles silently rage as the enemy attempts to subvert the physician's license for his economic and political benefit.

For the enemy to be victorious, the physician must serve the enemy's economic and political needs in addition to the patient's medical needs. To be victorious, the enemy must accomplish two goals: (1) Gain control of the physician's income, and (2) gain control over the implementation of his license.

Attainment of these two goals *is* Socialized Medicine. These goals can be attained only at the expense of physician civil rights, an event which must be by forfeit since these civil rights are a matter of law.

If the enemy had a legal right to these goals, it would have been claimed long ago.

Control of physician's income is to occur in the office through the assignment mechanism while control of his license is to occur in the hospital under the euphemistic headings "Utilization Review" and "Delineation of Privileges," two items which can easily be used to determine who the physician can treat and how he can treat.

Utilization Review can easily be expanded to completely control "who, when, and where" while Delineation of Privileges can easily be expanded to totally control "how" a patient will be treated.

8
Federal Control—
How to Prevent It
in the Office

ASSIGNMENTS: HOW TO/HOW NOT TO

In the present third-party atmosphere, the issue most destructive to private practice is the misunderstood issue of assignments.

In the battle to preserve private practice, a most basic premise is that the physician's economic security must *not* become dependent on *terms dictated by third-party carriers.* Most physicians have allready allowed this to happen *by forfeit* through ignorance of assignment law, primarily through ignorance of how to take assignments on Medicare patients.

There are two basic ways to insure payment of the physician's bill where insurance is involved, and thereby satisfy the intent of that insurance, i.e. payment of the doctor bill.

OPTION I.

Never take an assignment on a medicare form. Only when an assignment is taken on the Medicare form does the physician then enter into a contractual agreement to accept Medicare's determination of what his charge should be. (Read the reverse side of the Medicare form.) *To take a Medicare assignment need not bind one to its terms.* ON MEDICARE, OR OTHER INSURANCE-COVERED PATIENTS, TAKE YOUR ASSIGNMENT ON THE ENCLOSED SECTION VI APS OR UNDER

SIMILAR TERMS. *This leaves you completely free to charge the patient the balance whatever the third-party carrier pays.* This procedure alone will remove you from third-party economic control and from the role of being the source of the welfare which government says it is providing.

OPTION II.

Provide the patient with the amount of your bill only. When the bill has been paid by either cash, check, or promissory note, provide him with a completed Section VI APS marked "Paid." The patient then has adequate information to be reimbursed by his carrier. This second option circumvents the *necessity* of assignments in order to assure payment where insurance is involved, a situation fathered by negligent government which consistently refuses to enforce health insurance contracts which by law require "Proof of Loss" before the patient can receive payment from his carrier. Government allows the patient to use his doctor's bill which is actually notice of debt as proof of loss and thereby completely ignores reason, common sense, basic economics, and law. Only a *"paid"* doctor bill is legal proof of loss. Each physician, by Option II, has a legal right to do that which government refuses to do in order to assure the intent and economic theory of insurance contracts, and that is require a receipted bill as proof of loss where no assignment is taken.

If you choose the promissory note route, the following should be noted:

(a) You must report the notes as taxable income.
(b) You may charge interest on these notes since the patient no longer owes you a medical bill.
(c) The notes can be sold for a high percentage of their face value.
(d) Overdue notes can be collected through small claims court action.

The first option, taking assignments on your own terms, is the preferred course of action for all physicians *where they feel that payment for their services is in jeopardy.*

10084

DC-112-0 CARGILL'S—HOUSTON

ATTENDING PHYSICIAN'S STATEMENT

Name: _____ Age _____

HOSPITAL

Diagnosis: 1. _____ Admitted _____
          2. _____ Discharged _____
          3. _____
          4. _____

Disability due to: Illness _____ Accident on _____ Pregnancy _____ LMP _____

DATE	SERVICE RENDERED	CODE	CHARGES

Remarks: _____ _____ M.D.
(SIGNATURE)

_____ M.D.
(TYPED OR PRINTED NAME)

427 W. 20th Street
Houston, Texas 77008

PATIENT — INSURANCE INFORMATION

_____
(INSURANCE COMPANY AGENCY)

(POLICY NO. OR SOCIAL SECURITY NO.)

_____
(NAME OF INSURED)

_____
(EMPLOYER)

_____
(ADDRESS OF INSURED)

_____
(RELATIONSHIP OF PATIENT TO INSURED)

Date _____ Signature _____

ASSIGNMENT OF INSURANCE BENEFITS

PATIENT _____ GROUP # _____ POLICY # _____
CERTIFICATE # _____ MEDICARE # _____ MEDICAIDE # _____
I hereby authorize and direct the _____ to pay directly to _____
all benefits due me, if any, by reason of services described in the statements rendered, and as provided for in the above policy contract with the aforementioned insurance company. I will pay, at Houston, Texas, for all such charges incurred or for all charges in excess of whatever sums may be paid by the insurance company above mentioned.

SIGNATURE OF INSURED/PATIENT/AGENT   DATE

WITNESS
I hereby accept assignment of the benefits provided in this patient's policy.

ATTENDING PHYSICIAN

Constitutional lawyer ←

Gloria T. Svanas

Counsellor at Law

1813 East Eighth Street - Odessa, Texas 79761

915 337-1568

November 24, 1976   21

Dr. Ben B. White
Section VI Association
427 West 20th Street
Houston, Texas 77008

Doctor!
This is the most
important letter you will ever read!

Dear Dr. White:

        Based on a research of the applicable statutes, it is
my opinion that the Medicare program is simply an insurance
program funded by the United States through the Social Security
program. The contractural relationship between the government
and the potential patient is evidenced by the payment of premiums
by the insured to secure coverage under the Health Insurance Plan.
The government approved form Request for Medicare Payment specifically provides for completion by the patient and direct payment to
the patient upon the receipt of the form completed by the patient
only. The only way the Doctor becomes a party to the contract is if
the Doctor under Item 12 accepts the assignment and "agrees to accept
the charge determination of the Medicare carrier as the full charge
for covered services". The use of the language "covered" services
and the concluding instructions that the patient is "responsible
for the deductible, coinsurance and non-covered services" again
reiterate the fact that the Doctor is not a party to the contract.
Obviously, the right of the patient to be paid by attaching the
itemized bill from the Doctor exemplifies the fact that the Doctor
is not a party to the Contract nor is payment to the Doctor part
of the coverage by Medicare.

        Certainly, the Doctor should not subject his fees to the
"covered" services as determined by lay personnel. The Doctor is
entitled to the assignment of any insurance benefits and if they
should happen to include Medicare or Medicaid then the submitted form
of assignment of insurance benefits as part of the attending physician's
statement is the proper form for the Doctor to use to prevent his
charges from being subjected to the lay review. Obviously, once
the patient is well then the necessity for the services in the
eyes of the patient is greatly lessened. Furthermore, the Doctor
should be treating the patient to the extent of his ability based

Dr. Ben B. White
Page Two
November 24, 1976

* on the needs of the patient without regard to the limitations on the payment by reason of any insurance coverage that the patient might choose to purchase.

* Utilization review or recertification is an unenforceable third party requirement totally separate from the legal obligation of the insurer to pay the Request for Medicare Payment. Otherwise,
* the utilization review or recertification would constitute federal interference in the practice of medicine or the manner in which medical services are provided or compensation of any person providing
* health services as prohibited by Title 18 of the Social Security Act.

* It is my opinion that the physician has no duty to comply with any of the conditions of the Request for Medicare Payment unless he checks and signs Item 12 of the Medicare form stating that he accepts the assignment.

* Payments for the hospital bill by HEW or any other agency funded by the health insurance laws would be a separate contract between the patient and the insurer subject to the proof of the claim by the hospital. Any requirement for utilization review by the doctors practicing at the hospital as a condition precedent to
* the payment of the hospital bill would constitute supervision or control by a federal officer or employee over the manner in which medical services are provided. Furthermore, such requirement of
* utilization review is an attempt to illegally exercise supervision or control over the administration or operation of the hospital also prohibited by 42 U.S.C. §1801.

* Obviously, each Doctor must assert his constitutional right in the practice of medicine against the profit seeking compulsion by the hospital administration. The physician's sole
* duty is owed to the patient. The physician must exercise constant guard against any encroachment of his constitutional rights. A terminal slip would be the execution of an Application to practice in a hospital if the Application waives the physician's rights as
* an independent contractor or accepts the control by the hospital
* governing body of his practice of medicine.

A terrifying analogy can be made to the integration laws passed by Congress which specifically prohibit any forced busing to comply with the law, but the Federal Courts have judicially imposed forced busing and unfortunately, the affected citizens were not diligent enough to stop this illegal operation.

Respectfully submitted,

(Mrs.) Gloria T. Svanas

GTS/mat

Enclosure

THE MEDICARE CONSPIRACY

Mr. Thomas M. Tierney, Director
Bureau of Health Insurance
Social Security Administration
Baltimore, Maryland 21235

Re: The Medicare Conspiracy

Dear Mr. Tierney:

The law of assignment is well established in this country under the law of contract. It is the intent of Section VI that all physicians become aware of their constitutional legal rights in this matter. It is realized that a separate form may be a burden for the intermediaries but it is also realized that this burden can be relieved if Medicare will cease its efforts to violate inherent physician civil rights by the subversive methods it presently employs. If Medicare places on its forms the assignment terms to which physicians have a right, it may well be that all physicians would be willing to use the Medicare form. At present, the evidence indicates a concerted conspiracy on the part of HEW-Blue Cross-Blue Shield to violate inherent physician civil rights in this matter, evidence which indicates intent to mislead not only by a "Conspiracy of Silence" about what physicians' legal rights are but also to actively deny them of their civil rights by gross disregard for the assignment law of this land, and this is being done by an agency which is bound to uphold the law.

This conspiracy, this disregard for physician civil rights, this disregard for long established law will not be unchallenged.

Yours sincerely,
BEN B. WHITE, M.D.

DEPARTMENT OF HEALTH, EDUCATION, AND WELFARE
· SOCIAL SECURITY ADMINISTRATION
BALTIMORE, MARYLAND 21235

REFER TO: **NOV 30 1976**
IHI-631

Ben B. White, M.D.
Section VI Association
427 West 20th Street
Houston, Texas   77008

Dear Dr. White:

·This is in further response to your letters to the Secretary and the
Commissioner concerning the Medicare program.

We are not sure what you mean in stating that the doctrine of "fair play"
requires that Medicare advise all physicians of their legal options in the
matter of Medicare assignments nor in suggesting that Medicare is subverting
the rights of physicians through a "conspiracy of silence" and active violation of the law of assignment. The only statutory reference to assignment
in respect to physicians is in Section 1842(b)(3)(B)(ii). The substance
of this statutory reference is that physicians have the option of accepting
their patient's assignment of Medicare payment whereupon the Medicare payment
may be made directly to the physician under the condition that he accept
the Medicare determination of "reasonable charge" as his total charge for
the service or services for which he accepts assignment.

Medicare, through a number of informational issuances, has advised both
physicians and beneficiaries of this provision of law pointing out to both
parties that assignment is a mutual agreement between the physician and
the patient and that neither party is obligated by law to enter into such
an assignment agreement.

If you could be more specific about your allegations, we would be glad to
respond in more detail.

Sincerely yours,

· Thomas M. Tierney, Director
Bureau of Health Insurance .

Mr. Thomas M. Tierney, Director
Bureau of Health Insurance
Social Security Administration
Baltimore, Maryland 21235

Re: IHI-631

Dear Mr. Tierney:

May I express my appreciation for your letter of 30 November 76.

As an "Insurance Program" by name, definition, purpose, financing, participation, implementation, and therefore "Law," PL 89-97 is a contractual relationship between Government (HEW), intermediaries, certain persons age sixty-five years and over, and certain hospitals. The contractual nature is alluded to innumerable times. The word "Contract" or its equivalent appears ten times on the one page 310 which contains the referenced Section 1842 (b) (3) (B) (ii). The legal nature of such contractual relationships is that all parties are voluntary participants under terms and conditions of their choosing. This is how the concept of "freedom," which is designated legally as "Independent Contractor," is implemented according to the purpose of our Constitution, our government, as stated in the Preamble. Since physicians do not pay any premiums, did not sign any agreements and had nothing to do with the terms of PL 89-97, they owe no duty therein and are owed no duty thereby. Any participation by physicians is voluntary according to their constitutional rights whether that volition be informed or uninformed.

We are well aware of Sections 1801, 1814 (a) and 1842 (b) (3) (B) (ii) and consider Sections 1801 and 1814 (a) to be manifestations of congressional awareness of and recognition of the physicians legal rights. (Physicians, however, have not been properly informed of the legal meaning of these sections in-so-far as Utilization Review is concerned. It is very unlikely that HEW officials are aware of this either). But Section 1842 (b) (3) (B) (ii) is an attempt by the authors of this bill and therefore Congress-HEW to contract for the services of the physicians without their educated consent, a condition, the satisfaction of which can be legally achieved only by physician forfeit by virtue of ignorance of civil rights under the Thirteenth Amendment.

Under basic Contract Law, the physician is free to contract with his patient on his own terms. If the patient desires to assign his Medicare rights (benefits) to the physician, that physician is free to take the assignment on his own terms, i.e., to hold the patient responsible for the balance of what Medicare pays. Medicare can determine if its benefits are assignable or not but there is nothing in law or ethics that requires the physician to take assignment according to terms dictated by the federal government. It is recognized, of course, that through ignorance of assignment law, the physician can forfeit that constitutional right and that is why we hold HEW in contempt; contempt for unfairness, contempt for a "conspiracy of silence" since in the face of repeated efforts to point out this basic law, both HEW and BC-BS have not only exerted no effort to inform physicians of these points but have exerted efforts to subvert these rights. *Instances where BC-BS-HEW have, by devious mechanisms, violated these constitutional rights can be documented.* The day seems to be approaching when this documentation along with other gross efforts to violate physician-civil rights at the hospital staff level will see if the federal judicial process can expose this sickening disregard for physician-civil rights and the equally sickening ignorance of the economic mechanics at issue in both the Medicare and Medicaid programs.

> Yours sincerely,
> BEN B. WHITE, M.D.

"Medicare Assignments, Continued"

Section 1842 (b) (3) (B) (ii) of PL 89-97 states in essence that if a physician takes assignment on a Medicare patient, he must accept the government's determination of the amount of payment as payment in full. These terms are hidden in the printed material on the back of the Medicare form. If a physician completes this form, he, at the point of signature, enters into a contractual agreement with the government to accept those terms. There has been no violation of his Civil Right; he has just forfeited his Civil Right and has no cause to complain.

Previous pages have shown that physicians, as Independent Contractors under the Constitution, are free to take assignment on their own terms, and have illustrated how to do so. Section 1801 (a) provides for this. Section 1842 (b) (3) (B) (ii) is in violation of Section 1801 (a).
Many of these assignments, as recommended, have been received by Blue Cross-Blue Shield-Medicare and Medicare has refused to honor them. At this point, by this refusal to honor a duly executed assignment contract, Medicare violates physician Civil Rights. These physicians now have a cause of action against Medicare for Breach of Contract. But the individual physician is not financially able to tackle Uncle Sam and there is no organization to which he can turn for legal and financial aid to do so. The following is therefore suggested:

(1) Take the Medicare assignment on the regular Medicare form.

(2) At the block for physician's signature, sign and type this statement on each claim form "See attached Protest."

(3) By either a stamp on the form, or firmly attached to the form apply this statement, "I protest, as a violation of my civil right, being forced to take assignment under terms not of my free choice." _____ M.D. Date
_____.

(4) Once an assignment is taken, you are responsible for seeing that it is mailed.

(5) Notify all your Medicare patients that they will be charged the balance of what Medicare pays; bill and collect that balance.

(6) If Medicare can ignore your duly executed assignment terms, you can ignore theirs.

(7) Medicare will then be forced to either let the matter rest or file suit against the physicians who do this and the necessary judicial clarification will then be obtained.

Request for Additional Information

Dear (Patient):

Enclosed is a copy of a request for information received from Medicare. This information is not ordinarily requested by other carriers and is not furnished routinely by this office. To do so requires additional clerical effort and expense. My charge to Medicare for this additional clerical time and effort is $20.00, paid in advance. Thus far, Medicare has not honored bills for those additional services and the information will not therefore be provided. My office will not accept payment from you for that service.

When Medicare sees fit to prepay for the efforts it desires of my office personnel, the information will be provided.

Should Medicare continue to withhold funds from you under your Medicare contract or should it deduct the cost of this additional information from their payments, I strongly encourage you to complain to your Congressman.

Yours sincerely,
BEN B. WHITE, M.D.

cc: Medicare

DEPARTMENT OF HEALTH, EDUCATION, AND WELFARE
SOCIAL SECURITY ADMINISTRATION
BALTIMORE, MARYLAND 21235

REFER TO:
IHI-631

FEB 2 1977

Ben B. White, M.D.
Section VI Association
427 West 20th Street
Houston, Texas 77008

Dear Dr. White:

This is in further reply to your letters about the Medicare program.

Your most recent letter asserts that "If the patient desires to assign his Medicare rights (benefits) to the physician, that physician is free to take the assignment on his own terms; i.e., to hold the patient responsible for the balance of what Medicare pays." That is simply not correct and it would be regrettable if you continue to disseminate such misrepresentation in the face of the legal advice you have received from Mrs. Gloria T. Svanas, Counsellor at Law, in her letter to you dated November 24, 1976. She has, in this respect, advised you quite correctly when she states, in the second full paragraph on the second page, "It is my opinion that the physician has no duty to comply with any of the conditions of the Request for Medicare Payment unless (underlining ours) he checks and signs item 12 of the Medicare form stating that he accepts the assignment."

Clearly, what Mrs. Svanas is advising you is precisely what I tried to convey to you in my letter of November 30, 1976, that under Title 18, Section 1842(b)(3)(B)(ii), assignment under the Medicare program while wholly voluntary for both the patient and the physician, constitutes an acceptance by the physician of the payment conditions described on the Request for Medicare Payment if he confirms such acceptance by checking block 12 of that form. He is under no compulsion to do so, and we believe we have made this abundantly clear in our extensive informational activities directed to physicians.

As your lawyer has advised you, if the physician voluntarily accepts assignment, by checking block 12, he is then contractually bound to accept the conditions of payment clearly defined on the Request for Medicare payment.

Sincerely yours,

Thomas M. Tierney

Thomas M. Tierney, Director
Bureau of Health Insurance

I firmly believe that the director's letter is a delaying tactic, because he well knows what the issue is. No one denies what he says here, but he completely avoids the issue.

MOISTEN TO SEAL

MEDICARE PART B GROUP MEDICAL & SURGICAL SERVICE
P O BOX 22147, TEXAS 75222

00-6-329-363-02   **3**
PHONE AREA CODE 214/741-8864

IN ORDER TO PROCESS THE MEDICARE CLAIM RECEIVED ON **11/24/76** ADDITIONAL INFORMATION IS NEEDED.
PLEASE INDICATE ANSWERS IN SPACE PROVIDED BELOW EACH QUESTION, THEN FOLD AS INDICATED ON REVERSE AND RETURN.

DELAY NOTICE - BENJAMIN B WHITE   MD   SEE A AND C ON BACK.

DATE: **12-22-76**
RE:
77009   HI CLAIM NO. **445-03-3610-A**
ICN NUMBER.

1. INDICATE EXACT DATES OF HOSPITAL VISITS AND CHARGE PER VISIT FOR $150.00

2. INDICATE TYPE AND DOSAGE OF INJECTION ADMINISTERED ON OCT. 12, 1976 FOR $6.00,
INDICATE SPECIFIC DIAGNOSIS FOR EACH INJECTION.

3. INDICATE TYPE AND DOSAGE OF INJECTION ADMINISTERED ON OCT. 15, 1976 FOR $6.00,
INDICATE SPECIFIC DIAGNOSIS FOR EACH INJECTION.

This form also serves as a subtle effort to control their license drugs by promising to pay for drugs or procedures "they" disapprove of with.

If you do not supply this information because you sign this form you then "B" at that point agree to conditions "B" on the reverse side. BW

A LEGIBLE AND COMPLETE CLAIM IS THE FIRST STEP TOWARDS PROMPT AND ACCURATE SERVICE.

		OFFICE USE ONLY								

CONTROL # 00-6-329-363-02   6   DIGIT   CLERK

HIC (1)	CLM TYPE (2)	CLERK					
445033610A	P	X51B		1 OF 1 - 04			A00.

FIRST NAME (1)	INT (2)	LAST NAME (3)	SEX (4)	REL(5)	ASG(6) OS(7)	DIAG (8)	INTERFACE (9)
			M	N	N 2		A01.

BENEFICIARY STREET ADDRESS (1)
1138 LUZON   A02.

BENEFICIARY-CITY-STATE (1)	ZIP CODE (2)	CITY (3)	PROVIDER (4)	TOTAL CHARGES (5)	PATIENT-PAID (6)
HOUSTON TX	77009			016200	000000

A03.

ACIN	NAME(2)	PROVIDER(S)	SVC DTE(4)	PL(5)	T(.6)	PROC(7)	M/S(8)	CODE(9)			
P6	HO	805012	$24	IH	1	9019	010	015000	D	01	04
P6	HO	805012	101276	O	1	$32	010	000600	D	02	07
P6	HO	805012	101576	O	1	$32	010	000600	D	03	07
									D	.	.
									D	.	.
									D	.	.
									D	.	.
									D	.	.

NOTICE TO BENEFICIARY ONLY

Collection and Use of Medicare Information

We are authorized by the Social Security Administration to ask you for information needed in the administration of the Medicare program. Social Security's authority to collect information is in section 205(a), 1872 and 1875 of the Social Security Act, as amended.

The information we obtain to complete your Medicare claim is used to identify you and to determine your eligibility. It is also used to decide if the services and supplies you received are covered by Medicare and to insure that proper payment is made.

The information may also be given to other providers of services, carriers, intermediaries, medical review boards and other organizations as necessary to administer the Medicare program. For example, it may be necessary to disclose information about the Medicare benefits you have used to a hospital or doctor.

With one exception, which is discussed below, there are no penalties under Social Security law for refusing to supply information. However, failure to furnish information regarding the medical services rendered or the amount charged would prevent payment of the claim. Failure to furnish any other information, such as name or claim number, would delay payment of the claim.

If you are being treated for a work related injury, it is mandatory that you tell us so we can determine whether Workmen's Compensation will pay for the treatment. Section 1877 (a)(3) of the Social Security Act provides criminal penalties for withholding this information. (Please do not correspond with Medicare _unless_ you are being treated for a work related injury.)

──────────── SECOND FOLD ────────────

MEDICARE
GROUP MEDICAL & SURGICAL SERVICE
P.O. BOX 22147
DALLAS, TEXAS 75222

ATTENTION: DEVELOPMENT UNIT

──────────── FIRST FOLD ────────────

NOTES

Notes apply only when referenced from the front of this letter.

A. An initial letter requesting this information was sent to the provider indicated 18 days ago. Another letter has been sent to the provider at the same time as this letter. An accurate determination cannot be made on this claim until this information is received. If you can obtain this, be sure to return this letter along with the information or ask the provider to do so.

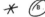

B. By signing this letter in the space indicated on the front, you are agreeing to accept assignment and will accept the charge determination of the Medicare carrier as the full charge.

C. If the requested information is not received within 21 days, this claim will have to be adjudicated on the basis of the evidence on hand. This might result in a disallowance or a reduction in the payment allowed.

2670.000 · MB376

The Medicaid Abuse Detection Manual

Dear Doctor:

In regard to the "Examiner's Guide for Medicaid Abuse Detection"—this is a beautiful but appalling demonstration of why it is so essential that physicians be aware of certain legal issues, their civil rights, with regard to Medicaid and Medicare.

The real crime is the monumental government stupidity regarding the free enterprise economics of health care.

It is impossible to police a program in which the provider of funds (HEW) plants the money tree in the front yard of both the "recipient of services" and the "provider of services" and says, "Here it is, boys, but *please* don't use it unless you really need it." A government that stupid deserves to be defrauded. This is to place absolute faith in the integrity of mankind and to deny totally the need for government as a mechanism for policing the economy of human association with the resulting creation of such problems as to require the creation of a massive bureaucracy to attempt to police those problems which would be non-existent if the very simple free enterprise approach had been used and the end result being that this new bureaucracy cannot succeed but like a Giant Blind Octopus which doesn't know what it is, why it is, or where it is, but only that it is hungry, will thrash around feeding on the civil rights of the populace under the false impression that what is good for its needs is good for the populace with the ultimate end result being destruction of the economy, the civil rights, and the product concerned.

Can you imagine the success one would have paying for all groceries and depending on the grocery store owner to keep people either out of the store or keep them from buying groceries "they don't need." It cannot be done that way. The laws of nature apply to economics, too, and just as birds can't fly under water and fish can't swim in the air, neither can the expenditure of funds be policed by those who benefit from those funds.

The individual is composed of two parts: (1) the desire for service, and (2) the ability to pay for service.

His ability to pay is the economic ballast, the policing action, against his desire. When another party assumes the economic duty, then that party must exercise any policing action against the one from whom he has taken that responsibility, against the desire for service, rather than against the provider of the service. It's like eating soup with a fork, writing books of regulations on how to hold the fork differently or squeeze it harder or threatening the one holding the fork. They just won't work. But that, my dear doctor, is the Medicaid program and "The Examiner's Guide for Medicaid Abuse Detection."

Yours sincerely,
BEN B. WHITE, M.D.

9
Federal Control—
How to Prevent It
in the Hospital

HOSPITAL CONTROL OF PHYSICIANS

Dear Doctor:

About 1970, the American College of Hospital Administrators sponsored several seminars apparently developed and conducted by an attorney, whose name will be withheld, attended by representatives of AHA, JCAH, and HEW in addition to local administrators and select personnel and concerning the general subject: "How can the hospitals legally gain complete control of the medical staffs." These seminars were held in various cities, were well attended and guarded to prevent attendance by "undesirable" persons.

It is assumed that it became apparent to this organization that the only way control of physicians can occur legally is by forfeit on the part of physicians. It was necessary therefore to contrive a mechanism at the Hospital Board of Governors—JCAH relationship level through which this control could be accomplished through physician forfeit by virtue of his ignorance of basic constitutional rights as a physician staff member.

The attorney who apparently began this subtle effort years ago with the American College of Hospital Administrators is now a staff member of the Joint Commission on Accreditation of Hospitals. (He departed JCAH as of December, 1975, but is officed nearby.)

It seems to be a reasonable conclusion that the general effort to revise Hospital Staff Constitution and By-Law is the result of those efforts, efforts directed towards legal control of physicians by the AHA-JCAH-HEW complex, such control to be obtained through physician ignorance, physician forfeit of certain basic constitutional rights.

You are therefore urged to review the enclosed comments and give extremely careful consideration to all proposals which would change your staff Constitution and By-Law as a "condition for accreditation."

Yours sincerely,
BEN B. WHITE, M.D.

UTILIZATION REVIEW VS. PEER REVIEW

Dear Doctor:

One of our major problems is getting physicians to understand the difference between *legal duty* and *ethical duty*. Therein lies the confusion about "Utilization Review" which is really "Utilization Curtailment." The following illustration is helpful:

An insurance company (IC) sells a patient (P) a life preserver, but P says, "I don't want to carry it with me, just get it to me when I really need it." We will call the doctor (Dr.) a lifeguard. Dr. is strolling along the beach when he hears a distress call from P who he sees apparently drowning. Dr. has an *ethical* duty to do what he is trained to do but he has no *legal* duty to make the rescue attempt. It is Dr.'s choice. If Dr. chooses to make the attempt, he has a *legal* duty to do so with reasonable care and skill. Dr. starts to swim out. IC is observing because of its *economic* interest. As you (Dr.) start to swim, IC jumps on your back, (the back of ethics) for a free ride to see if a life preserver is really needed and wants Dr. to certify to that effect. IC is using your license, your ability for its economic interests. If you went out in a boat and IC jumped in for a free ride, that is the third party using your history, Physical, Operative Notes, Progress Notes—*all your personal property*—for its *economic* benefit. I say make IC swim out and make its own assessments. (True peer review is another lifeguard (Dr.) observing your abilities, another lifeguard who has no economic interest in the situation.) This may not sound too bad on the surface if Dr. understands he has no *legal* duty to give IC the free ride. But IC is a larger party than Dr. with a very tangible economic interest. If Dr. is not aware of his rights relative to IC, then he will eventually succumb to all kinds of rules and regulations concerning his own qualifications, who he can rescue, when, where, and how, re-qualification, etc., all to protect the *economic* interests of IC under the cloak of ethics and all because of Dr.'s failure to understand that he has no *legal* duty to provide the free ride (Utilization Review) in the first place, nor does he have the *legal* duty to provide access to his personal property by IC for IC's use in making that determination.

Yours sincerely,
Ben B. White, M.D.

MEDICAL STAFF CONSTITUTION AND BY-LAWS

In these trying times of overt and subtle attempts by the federal government to gain control of private practitioners, it is essential that these practitioners become aware of the methods used to gain such control. It is essential they understand the sequence of events which opened the door for selfish third party intervention in medical practice.

There are two prerequisites for federal control. (1) In the office, the *physician's income is to be controlled* by controlling his charges through his ignorance of assignment law; and (2) in the hospital, *his license is to be controlled* through his subjugation to rules established by HEW acting for economic reasons through JCAH and JCAH overreacting to certain events to protect the economic interests of the hospital. Control of income and control of license by third parties is *socialized medicine*.

This communication concerns the latter issues and was precipitated by the proposed Medical Staff Constitution and By-Law changes.

Before proceeding further it should be stated and it must be recognized that a constitution and by-law, just as the U.S. Constitution and its Amendments, is the written manifestation of the independence of the organization concerned. It is a two-edged sword which serves not only as a guide for duties to be performed to achieve the purpose of the organization but also to protect from forced performance in areas not concerned with the purposes of the organization.

It is recognized that changes are needed but any changes which occur must promote, support, and improve on the fact that physicians are independent contractors who, for ethical reasons, organize to protect the public interest insofar as medical care is concerned and thereby must remain free and independent of third-party economic interests less economizing policies be transferred to patients as economizing medical care. Just because change is indicated, we must not overreact selfishly and unilaterally as AHA and JCAH have done because of fear induced by unfortunate events in related areas of social encounter. For a "joint" organization, the JCAH certainly does not exhibit the concern for the rights of the physician it should but rather places all emphasis on patient's, hospital's, and third-party interests while relegating physicians to the category of hired help.

For specific comments on the proposed changes: (*See* By-Laws below)

ITEM 1.

It is unethical and illegal for the medical staff to subject itself to the Constitution and By-Law of a corporate entity. The reason for this is that corporations only have tangible economic (legal) interests in patient care while physicians alone are responsible for the intangible quality of medical care. The law recognized this by the Medical Practice Act. Section VI of the Code of Ethics recognizes this.

ITEM 2.

This "whereas" contains the basic false premise on which the major changes are founded, the same false premise which lost the Darling case, a case which instilled fear into the JCAH and AHA and resulted in marked overreaction, a case which has since been relegated to the oblivion which it so rightly deserved. The governing body cannot delegate the responsibility for quality of care to the medical staff. The governing body has never had that responsibility. Quality of care is the legal responsibility of physicians as a matter of law whether it be in his office, hospital or wherever. It is also twisted logic to say "we delegate it; it is your responsibility, but in the long run we are responsible." *(Item 3.)*

ITEM 4.

"Cooperative efforts" is another term for "liaison" which is the method used by separate legal entities to arrive at satisfactory conclusions for mutual problems without interfering with or infringing upon each other's legal rights. This phrase is therefore a proper recognition of the staff's independence, a position which is basically opposed by JCAH and thereby again demonstrates the confused state of that organization. (See below *Items 16, 17,* and *18.*)

ITEM 5.

As for the "hospital's obligation" to its patients, that does not, because of lack of qualification, include responsibility for policing quality of care. If the hospital were legally responsible for medical care, then it would have the correlative duty of hiring, supervising and dictating to licensed physicians otherwise it would be negligent in its duties. This quite obviously cannot be.

ITEM 6.

Physicians and dentists should have separate staff organizations to illustrate their independence. The JCAH should require this.

ITEM 7.

Licensing and limitation of license is a function of the state, a point which must be kept in mind when considering such issues as "Delineation of Privileges."

ITEM 8.

This may seem to be a minor point when in actuality it is a very important point. Physicians do not admit patients. Only the hospital admits and dismisses and this has significant legal implications. Physicians only recommend.

ITEM 9.

Again the dental staff should declare its autonomy by establishing its own constitution and by-law.

ITEM 10.

Again, it is recognized that changes are needed in the matter of physician qualifications, but it is also true that attempts to correct faults in isolated and haphazard fashion outside the realm of organized medicine is to deny the need for organized medicine. It will result in confusion, lack of uniformity, further fragmentation, friction, and law suits and will in general cause much more harm than good to the cause of private practice and quality care. It is not only dangerous from a legal viewpoint but is an illegal attempt by those without the authority to limit the unlimited license granted by the state. Such limitation is a function of the state and efforts to do so should be directed through organized medicine to the State Board if fairness, uniformity, unanimity and effectiveness are to be achieved. It seems reasonable that it is time that license be granted for the specific field of practice to be entered after completion of a prescribed course of training.

ITEM 11.

This is a good statement, but what does it mean? It is the *right* of an independent staff to *initiate rules for self-government* and not be dictated by other organizations.

ITEM 12.

Also good because again it provides for that "liaison" which is the method used by separate legal entities to reach satisfactory solutions for mutual problems. This item's presence again is a sign of the confusion on the part of JCAH on the issues of legal rights, legal duty and ethical duty.

ITEM 13.

Again, very good to state that the Constitution and By-Law cannot require members to perform functions not pertinent to patient care. This being so, there is no reason whatever to subjugate the members to the rules of an organization whose legal concern and primary interest is economic and who has a public interest in quality of medical care but no duty in quality of medical care.

ITEM 14.

A medical staff must investigate candidates through the medical society. This is a primary reason for both the medical organization and the medical staff organization. To fail to require medical society membership as a prerequisite for staff membership is to deprive the staff of a way to accomplish its purpose and to deny the need for organized medicine and its Code of Ethics because it is only on the basis of this membership, this Code of Ethics that the staff has the authority or ability to police its members.

ITEMS 16, 17, 18.

The purpose of the Thirteenth Amendment is to designate all individual members of society as independent contractors. This might be considered to be the legal designation of freedom or liberty. With this designation is the freedom to associate on terms of one's own choosing A medical staff is an independent organization of independent individuals organized for the *ethical* purpose of defending the public interest in the matter of medical care. The hospital on the other hand is a legal organization operating for economic reasons. These are two separate legal entities. Section VI of the AMA Code of Ethics requires that the medical staff operate independently of other organizations. Law does not require physicians to place themselves subject to the rules and regulations of corporate entities and in fact provides that this not be done. *As an independent organization, a medical staff has the legal right to have final authority on the matter of membership.* It can and has in the past forfeited this right but to do so is to violate both the law and the Code of Ethics. The JCAH cannot require as a condition for accreditation in an ethical organization that a physician forfeit any of his Civil Rights. To do so deprives that physician of due process.

ITEM 19.

It is agreed that there is a need for continuing education but this is a proper function of organized medicine, a function which it continues to avoid as an ethical requirement. But to act in this manner, to limit the exercise of one's license, is to perform a legal act under the cloak of ethics and cannot produce a desirable result. On the contrary, it will invite further legal requirements under the guise of ethics (Utilization Review). The staff must recognize that its duty is to judge the quality of the implementation of that unlimited license, a retrospective judgment, which is an ethical evaluation rather than to attempt prejudgment or limitation of license which is a legal act. This basic idea is recognized in Item 20, a statement which holds true for this license in general.

Summary and Conclusion

Years ago, before the science of medicine had advanced to its present state, there were areas of concern. The JCAH was the result of this concern, this feeling that the public needed better protection in the field of medical care. This was a time of almost no specialization, a time when the doctor-patient relationship existed by mutual trust rather than by law. The legal duties and rights of the parties were not so well defined as now.

JCAH was an admirable venture just as organized medicine is. But JCAH like organized medicine did not occur from *legal duty* but rather ethical duty. The JCAH like *Good Housekeeping* merely says to the ublic, "Here is a hospital and medical staff which we have judged as providing a 'fair deal' for those who use their facilities and services."

The JCAH provides no money to patients and takes no money from them. Its interest is not economic, i.e., legal or political. Its interest is ethical.

But the insurance industry whose interest *is* economic or legal injected itself or its economic interest years ago by refusing to pay for services of a non-accredited hospital. So third-party economic interests were slipped in under the cloak of ethics and to this day all parties continue to be confused in this area, a confusion which is the basis of all our problems with third parties. This insurance industry position was not clarified at law, and finally after forty years, HEW, as another economic interest, has not only done the same thing but, in addition, is trying to force on doctors, through JCAH, rules and regulations which serve only to protect HEW's economic and political interests. On top of this, and because of a related social problem, the malpractice issue, the JCAH, an ethical organization, is trying to exercise legal power through license limitation and certain other dictates which are matters of law—not ethics—in order to protect the economic or legal interests of the hospital. By allowing this third-party influence to determine their conditions for accreditation, the JCAH has prostituted, defeated its original purpose and will now become a tool of the economic interests of the federal government just as has Blue Cross-Blue Shield.

If physicians cannot prevent that event, then it is time to up-date the purpose of the JCAH by abandoning it and forming separate accreditation organizations—one from the AMA to accredit the medical staff, one from the AHA to accredit the hospital plant and personnel, and one from the ANA to accredit the nursing staff because the public will still be in need of ethical protection, i.e., protection from both these primarily economic interests and incompetent physicians.

BY-LAWS OF THE MEDICAL STAFF
HEIGHTS HOSPITAL, HOUSTON, TEXAS
(PROPOSED BY JCAH)

WHEREAS, Heights Medical Center, Inc, is a *corporation (1)* organized under the laws of the State of Texas; and

WHEREAS, Its purpose is to serve as a general hospital providing patient care, education and research; and

WHEREAS, It is recognized that the *governing body has delegated (2)* to the medical staff the responsibility for the quality of medicare in the hospital and the medical staff must accept and discharge this responsibility, *subject to the ultimate authority (3)* of the hospital governing body, and that the *cooperative (4)* efforts of the medical staff, the administrator and the governing body are necessary to fulfill the *hospital's obligations (5)* to its patients; therefore, be it

RESOLVED, That the physicians and *dentists (6)* practicing in this hospital hereby organize themselves into a medical staff in conformity with these by-laws.

Definitions

1. The term "staff" and "medical" staff: mean all physicians holding *unlimited (7)* licenses, and duly licensed dentists who are privileged to attend patients in the hospital.

2. The term "governing body" means the board of directors of the hospital.
3. The term "executive committee" means the executive committee of the medical staff.
4. The term "president of the medical staff" is synonymous with chief of staff.
5. The term "administrator" means the individual appointed by the governing body to act in its behalf in the overall management of the hospital.
6. The term "practitioner" means appropriately licensed physicians and dentists.
7. The term "medical staff year" means the calendar year.
8. Specified professional personnel shall be defined as those professionals who assist members of the medical staff in the care of patients within the limits of their skills and experience. patients shall be *admitted only by physicians (8)* of the medical staff. *Dentists of the medical staff (9)* may also admit patients, but only with the concurrence of physicians of the medical staff.

Article I: Name

The name of this organization shall be the Medical Staff of Heights Hospital.

Article II: Purposes

The purposes of this organization are:
1. To provide that all patients admitted to or treated in any of the facilities, departments, or (?) of the hospital shall receive the best possible care;
2. To provide a high level of professional performance of all practitioners authorized to practice in the hospital through the appropriate *delineation (10)* of the clinical privileges that each practitioner may exercise in the hospital and through an ongoing review and evaluation of each practitioner's performance in the hospital;

3. To provide an appropriate educational setting that will maintain scientific standards and that will lead to continuous advancement in professional knowledge and skill;
4. To *initiate* and *maintain rules* and *regulations for self-government (11)* of the medical staff; and
5. To provide a means where issues concerning the medical staff and the hospital may *be discussed (12)* by the medical staff with the governing body and the administrator of the hospital.
6. The medical staff organization shall have no power to *require* a member of the staff to perform *functions not pertinent to patient medical care. (13)*

Article III: Medical Staff Membership

SECTION 1.   NATURE OF MEDICAL STAFF MEMBERSHIP

Membership on the medical staff of the hospital is a privilege which shall be extended only to professionally competent physicians and dentists holding unlimited licenses, who continuously meet the qualifications, standards and requirements set forth in these by-laws.

SECTION 2.   QUALIFICATIONS FOR MEMBERSHIP

a. Only practitioners licensed to practice in the State of Texas who can *document* their *background, experience, training and demonstrated competence,* their *adherence to the ethics of their profession (14)* their good reputation, and their ability to work with others with sufficient adequacy to assure the medical staff and the governing body that any patient treated by them in the hospital will be given a high quality of medical care, shall be qualified for membership on the medical staff. No physician or dentist shall be entitled to membership on the medical staff or to the exercise of particular clinical privileges in the hospital merely by virtue of the fact that he is duly licensed to practice medicine or dentistry in this or in any other state, or that he is a member of any professional organization, that he had in the past, or presently has, such privileges at another hospital, or that he had, in the past, such privileges or membership at this hospital.

b. Acceptance of membership on the medical staff shall constitute the staff *member's agreement* that he will strictly *abide by the Principles of Medical Ethics (14)* of the American Medical Association, by the Code of Ethics of the American Dental Association, by the Code of Ethics of the American Osteopathic Association, by the Code of Ethics of the Texas Medical Association, or by the Code of Ethics of the American College of Surgeons, whichever is applicable, as the same are amended from time to time and made a part of these by-laws.

c. No person shall be excluded from membership on the staff because of race, color, religion, sex or national origin. Acceptance of membership on the staff shall constitute the *staff member's agreement* that he will *admit* and treat *all patients (15)* on a completely non-discriminatory basis, without regard to race, color, religion, sex or national origin.

SECTION 3.   CONDITIONS AND DURATION OF APPOINTMENT

a. Initial *appointments* and *reappointments* to the medical staff *shall be made by the governing body. (16)* The governing body shall act on appointments only after there has been a recommendation from the medical staff as provided in these by-laws; provided that in the event of unwarranted delay on the part of the medical staff, the governing body may act without such recommendation on the basis of documented evidence of the applicant's or staff member's professional and ethical qualifications obtained from reliable sources other than the medical staff. However, in no case shall the Board of Trustees take action on an application, refuse to renew an appointment or cancel an appointment, previously made, without conference with the staff or its representative.

b. Initial appointments shall be for a period extending to the end of the current medical staff year of the hospital. Reappointments shall be for a period of not more than one medical staff year.

c. Appointment to the medical staff shall confer on the appointee only such *clinical privileges as have been granted by the (17)* governing body, in accordance with these by-laws.

d. Every application for staff appointment shall be signed by the applicant and shall contain the applicant's specific acknowledgment of every medical staff member's obligations to provide continuous care and supervision of his patients, *to abide by the by-laws of the governing body (18)* and the medical staff by-laws, rules and regulations, to accept committee assignments and to accept consultation assignments.

Article VI: Clinical Privileges

SECTION 1.   DELINEATION OF CLINICAL PRIVILEGES *(19)*

a. Every practitioner practicing at this hospital by virtue of medical staff membership or otherwise shall, in connection with such practice, be entitled to exercise only those clinical privileges specifically granted to him by the governing body, upon the recommendation of the medical staff, except as provided in Sections 2 and 3 of this Article VI. In accordance with the provisions of Article XIV, Section 2, of these by-laws, the medical staff shall establish and amend, as necessary, rules and regulations governing the delineation of clinical privileges of its members.

b. Privileges granted to dentists shall be based on their training, experience, and demonstrated competence and judgment. The scope and extent of surgical procedures that each dentist may perform shall be delineated and granted in the same manner as all other surgical privileges. Surgical procedures performed by dentists shall be under the overall supervision of the chairman of the operating room committee. A dentist with hospital privileges may initiate the admission of a patient with the concurrence of a member of the medical staff, but no admission may be completed without such concurrence. All dental patients shall receive the same basic medical appraisal as patients admitted for other surgical procedures. The medical staff member concurring in a patient's admission assumes responsibility for the overall medical care of the patient, including the medical history and physical examination. When dental surgery is indicated, the member of the medical staff may assume supervision of the patient during the surgical procedure. *The nature and degree of his participation is a matter for his determination (20)* in each case within the general policy adopted by the medical staff governing the relationship and dual responsibility between the physician and the dentist. The dentist may write orders within the scope of his license as limited by the applicable statutes and the rules and regulations of the medical staff. The care of the dental patient is the dual responsibility of the dentist and the physician.

THE AHA-JCAH-HEW CONSPIRACY

Dear Doctor:

In the final analysis, the crux of the present Constitution and By-Law issue is that the goal of the AHA-JCAH-HEW complex is:

1. To protect the economic interests of HEW through committee limitation of the doctor's license to admit and discharge as he and his patient see fit (erroneously called "Utilization Review").
2. To protect the hospital economic interests in the field of liability by committee (staff) limitation of the unlimited license granted to the physician, and serve as the foundation for future expansion of control of "how" the physician exercises his license. The JCAH is to be the instrument through which these economic interests are protected as "Conditions for Accreditation."

Since both the JCAH and the medical staff were organized for ethical reasons, neither law nor ethics supports these efforts to protect economic interests; and therefore, any success by those parties to use the physician's license to protect their economic interests will be due to sacrifice by the physician of his legal rights.

Neither of these efforts is grounded in sound economics, cannot therefore be successful and will result in even greater future restrictions on the doctor as these fruitless efforts continue. It's like squeezing a fork harder to make it a better instrument with which to eat soup. The wrong principle is involved. It won't work and will eventually destroy the innocent fork for being unable to do that which it was not designed to do.

The U.S. Supreme Court in *"Doe* vs. *Bolton"* (1973) clearly states the doctor's legal position: "If a physician is licensed by the State, he is recognized by the State, he is capable of exercising acceptable clinical judgment. If he fails in this, professional censure and deprivation of his license are available remedies. *Required acquiescense by co-practitioners (Committees) has no rational connection with the patient's needs and unduly infringes on the physician's right to practice"* (emphasis added).

The excess verbiage about "due process" is a subterfuge to give physicians the psychological feeling that the Staff Constitution and By-Law has the trappings of law, i.e., a legal document rather than an ethical document and therefore anything therein is absolute and final. Due process is a matter of civil statute, not ethics, and need not be in the Constitution and By-Law except perhaps as a passing statement that the staff recognizes and intends to abide by all state and federal laws.

In essence, there is no need to revise the basic present Constitution and By-Law other than to delete certain items already there but certainly not to add anything.

The enclosed letter is therefore recommended.

Yours sincerely,
BEN B. WHITE, M.D.

Recommended Letter

Dr. John Porterfield
The Joint Commission on Accreditation of Hospitals
875 North Michigan Avenue
Chicago, Illinois 60611

Dear Dr. Porterfield:

The _____ Hospital Medical Staff is of the opinion that the purpose of organized medicine and an organized medical staff is ethical. That is, the organization exists to protect the public interest in an area in which the civil and criminal statutes cannot so protect. No law requires the existence of this staff organization. On the other hand, the hospital operates under license and charter and is governed by civil statutes. Its Constitution and By-Law, therefore, are not founded in ethics, but for the legal purposes of promoting and protecting the economic interest of that facility. We, therefore, have two separate organizations, one founded in ethics, and one founded on legalities. Section VI of the AMA Code of Ethics dictates that ethical considerations should not be subjected to legal or economic considerations. We therefore believe that it is unethical for the staff to subject itself to the Constitution and By-Law of the Board of Trustees of _____ Hospital. We also believe that it is illegal for the JCAH to require this as a condition for accreditation since it would be a violation of the individual staff member's civil rights.

We feel that it is absolutely necessary that this staff require membership in the local Harris County Medical Society as a condition for membership on the medical staff. Otherwise, we would have no mechanism available to conduct the policing duty required by ethics.

In addition, "Delineation of Privileges" is a euphemistic expression for "Limitation of License." Licensing and limitation of license is under the authority of the state. Neither the hospital nor the medical staff have the legal or ethical duty or authority to limit that license as a condition for the privilege of exercising that license. We feel that it is unlawful for the JCAH to require this as a condition for accreditation or for the staff to require it as a condition for membership.

We, therefore, will not accept these three recommendations by the JCAH as condition for accreditation and will take whatever action is necessary should accreditation be denied because of this action.

Yours sincerely,
President,_____Hospital Staff

HOSPITAL STAFF MEMBERSHIP

Dear Doctor:

Considerable confusion has existed at the judicial level and still exists at all other levels of society over the question of hospital or doctor responsibility for hospital patient injury. This confusion led to the infamous Darling decision which found the hospital liable for the acts of a staff member. Later judicial analysis cleared the air considerably by destroying the Darling decision. This eventual result was a certainty as the courts eventually pointed out that the physician as an independent contractor is solely responsible for the exercise of his license. But the situation which caused the confusion has not yet been corrected and remains therefore a potential source of difficulty for hospital and staff.

The confusion exists because for many years the staff, by forfeit, has allowed the hospital trustees to have final vote on staff membership. To have this duty implied that said trustees have a degree of legal authority over the member and therefore have a degree of responsibility for his actions when in fact no such legal conditions exist. The courts keep telling us, "You are independent contractors, so please act as such." As an organization of independent contractors the staff has the legal right to determine who its members will be and that vote is not subject to review, confirmation, or rejection by the trustees. We must exercise this right. It will aid greatly in clearing the air with regard to hospital-physician responsibility in many matters. Failure to exercise this right will cause serious consequences in the future as management and JCAH attempt to exert more control over the physician.

Sincerely yours,
BEN B. WHITE, M.D.

HOSPITAL RECORDS

This portion is a shot fired in anger at the legal profession and the judiciary for their total disregard for physicians as individuals with basic constitutional rights. This disregard is based on ignorance resulting from failure to carefully analyze that collection of paperwork called a "Hospital Medical Record." It is also a call for physicians to stand up and defend their civil rights rather than suffer defeat under the sword of forfeit.

The greatest obstacle which physicians face in their efforts to (1) establish a defense against third party encroachment into the practice of medicine and (2) preserve their own security and liberty as citizens is *ignorance* on the part of the legal profession and judiciary. This *ignorance* is evident when matters related to the practice of medicine arise which have no precedent and when issues regarding the practice of medicine or physicians' civil rights arise and are poorly defended because of failure of the legal profession to properly identify the issues. As in the field of malpractice, physicians have become clay pigeons trapped on the platform of medical practice which has been converted into a public shooting gallery by judicial and legislative negligence. We have no advocate in an adversary system.

First and foremost, the Hospital Chart should be divided *by physicians* into two parts: (1) The Hospital Chart and (2) the Attending Physician's Chart. This action should have been recommended by legal counsel long ago. Secondly, and of equal importance, is to understand that the History, Physical, Progress

Notes, Operative Report, Consultation, and Discharge Summary do not constitute the "Patient's Record." They are part of the "Physician's Record." As such it serves three purposes:

1. It is written manifestation of the physician's license and therefore is the legal manifestation of his competence as a physician, i.e., of his ability to use symptoms provided by the patient together with findings from his examination to reach a proper diagnosis on which to render appropriate therapy. The record contains language completely foreign to the patient and therefore is incapable of the patient's analysis. As the legal manifestation of the doctor's license, it is also the legal manifestation of his liability.

2. It is written to provide a means whereby other physicians of similar training can, with the physician's knowledge and consent, review his efforts and thereby fulfill the profession's ethical duty to maintain quality care for the public. This review is, as a matter of law, not subject to third-party review even under subpoena (Texas Revised Civil Statutes 4447 d Section 3).

3. It is written for future reference by the same or other physicians for the above purposes.

The Attending Physician's Record, by virtue of origination as the result of his acquired skill and knowledge and the exercise of the constitutional right of freedom of contract, represents *his* personal competence, contains *his* liability, and is therefore *his* personal property according to constitutional rights and protections established under the First, Fifth, Thirteenth, and Fourteenth Amendments, all judicial opinions thus far to the contrary notwithstanding.

The only uses a patient can possibly have for the Attending Physician's Chart is as a source of information for civil suits not related to the purpose of the chart or to search for reasons for a cause of action against the physician. The physician is under no duty to serve as a clerk, secretary, or corroborating source for the patient in such civil actions in the former instance and certainly under no duty to furnish information which could be used against him in the latter instance. To force the physician to submit these records in the first instance is a violation of the Thirteenth and Fourteenth Amendments and, in the latter instance, a violation of the Fifth Amendment. The patient remains in possession of any information he may need for such civil suits and any laboratory or radiological reports can be obtained from the Hospital Chart.

The attending physician is legally responsible only for diagnosis and medical description of treatment rendered and this responsibility extends only to the patient or such parties as have legal need to know.

Those parties have no authority to question or even peruse the matter in which a physician arrives at a diagnosis. The state licensed him to do that.

Since these records contain the physician's liability, the only duty he has to *anyone* insofar as completeness and accuracy of content is the duty to himself to protect his own interest insofar as his liability is concerned. The record is of no concern to anyone other than the previously mentioned Medical Staff Committee for purposes of internal policing of quality. He is advised to keep adequate and correct records to be used at his discretion for his own legal protection in any future litigation to which he is a party.

The physician is legally obligated not to divulge to any parties, without consent, any interpretations of the patient's symptoms and physical or laboratory findings. He is well within his right to state personal opinions or feelings about the patient and/or staff and/or hospital in this record without fear of publication because those personal feelings can and do influence the manner in which he practices. Whether they do or not, they are his personal responsibility and liability.

To hold that the Attending Physician's Chart is the property of the patient is erroneous. It shows gross and even malicious disregard for the rights of physicians and *must* be contested by *all physicians* all the way to the Supreme Court where undoubtedly right will prevail.

It would be well for physicians to exert their right in this matter by keeping the items which they author and/or sign separate from the Hospital Chart and remove those items to their office when the patient is dismissed.

The JCAH is not the physician's advocate.

The AMA has not been the physician's advocate.

The legal profession and the Judiciary have not done their duty towards physicians.

Physicians apparently will have to learn the law of Contract, Tort, and Personal Property in in order to be their own advocate not only in this matter but in many others.

A Clarification

Dr. John Porterfield
The Joint Commission on Accreditation of Hospitals
875 North Michigan Avenue
Chicago, Illinois 60611

Dear Dr. Porterfield:

It would be illogical for one to deny that changes are indicated in the hospital practice of medicine but such changes must not be restrictive in nature insofar as practitioner ability is concerned. Such changes should be directed toward improvement of practitioner ability. Quality of medical care, which is a proper concern of medical staffs and the JCAH, is not maintained or improved by harassment of, coercion of, or restrictions on practitioners but is determined by original training and continuing education of these practitioners. The issue of quality is an ethical issue. The JCAH, an ethical organization, must not therefore presume to become a legal body in an effort to correct certain deficiencies. If it does so, it will eventually forfeit its ethical position and thereby aid in depriving the public of quality control.

The specific issue to which I refer is the issue of "Delineation of Privileges." There will be minimal, if any, public benefit if different medical staffs in a haphazard manner attempt to restrict one another's license, but there is much to be gained by required levels of original and continuing education done in a standardized manner.

We are presented with an excellent opportunity to change the long entrenched concept of unlimited licensing for M.D.'s, a concept which is not compatible with present degrees of specialty training. Recommendations should be made by the AMA and the JCAH to the powers that be that licensing be changed from unlimited to limited. For instance, license should be granted to an M.D. to do general practice after completion of a prescribed three-year G.P. residency, or to a Neurosurgeon for Neurosurgery after the prescribed residency program. This would in essence delete the need for what JCAH is trying to accomplish through "Delineation of Privileges." The medical organization should then add an additional section to its Code of Ethics to the effect that "a physician shall remain abreast of current developments in his field of practice."

As stated in previous communication, licensing, or limitation of license, is a duty of the state. Any efforts to do so must originate there. To act otherwise is to deny this legitimate function of government and result in non-standardized guidelines which will cause confusion, friction and further social chaos.

It seems that the State Board of Medical Examiners should intervene in JCAH activities in this area before much more damage is done if JCAH does not voluntarily reconsider its position.

There are several other requirements for accreditation in which the JCAH is attempting to act in a legal area and thereby endangering the purpose of medical organizations and the JCAH.

Due process is a legal issue, a statutory issue. Due-process mechanics should not be included in the Constitution and By-Law of the medical staff, which is an ethical organization.

It is recognized that applicants and members of certain committees may need due-process guidelines but these guidelines should be furnished as a separate booklet compiled by the AMA legal department, and for convenience, made available on request to applicants, staff members, or members of the administrative staff. It should not be a requirement that these guidelines be in the staff Constitution and By-Law as a condition for accreditation except perhaps by reference.

One other item. Physicians are independent contractors under the Constitution. They voluntarily join an ethical organization, a medical staff, for the purpose of controlling quality as an ethical public duty. The hospital, through its Board of Trustees, is an economic entity, a legal entity, chartered under the civil statutes of the state. It is a corporation. A physician does not voluntarily join that corporation. It may be a violation of the Medical Practice Act if he does place himself subject to the dictates of that corporation's Constitution and By-Law. In my opinion, it is a violation of physician civil rights to be required to abide by the corporate Constitution and By-Law as a condition for accreditation, and certainly a violation of Section VI of the AMA Code of Ethics.

In my opinion, the State Attorney General's office should review this JCAH "condition for accreditation," should the JCAH refuse to withdraw this condition for accreditation.

Yours sincerely,
BEN B. WHITE, M.D.

10
Forewarned Is Forearmed

TEXAS MEDICAL FOUNDATION

Dear Doctor,

A letter to Texas physicians from the Texas Medical Foundation containing the remarks the Executive Director made in San Antonio on May 1, 1975, should alarm all physicians because it expresses a philosophy that means the demise of private practice if physicians fail to understand it.

That letter, sincere and well intended as it is, manifests ignorance of the purpose and meaning of Section VI of the AMA Code of Ethics; disregard for physicians' civil rights, and ignorance of both the free enterprise system and the mechanics of third-party efforts to control practitioners. It is filled with falsehoods and misleading terminology comparable to Wilbur Cohen's best deceptive efforts, a most disastrous and damning example of the ineptness of organized medicine's efforts to deal with third parties. The really sad part is that neither TMA (Texas Medical Association) nor TMF officials understand its implications. Were this not true, there would never have been a TMF. To state otherwise would be to accuse them of treason. The net result is the same, however, as the TMA effectively works through its "hatchet," the TMF, to aid in the demise of private practice.

For private practitioners to embrace the TMF is suicidal. The TMF is the Pied Piper to certain destruction, an unwitting Trojan horse. It recognizes as lost that which cannot be lost except by forfeit. It would forfeit that which must not be forfeited and then, under the euphemistic phrase "corporate agent," assume a Union-type posture through which it would "bargain" to regain that which it gave away, that which is not subject to diminution by political bargaining, that which is of ultimate importance in the battle to preserve private practice, namely, physician civil rights.

The private practice of medicine is not a "Group" or "Corporate" or "Foundation" activity. It is the individual application of special individual training, under license by the state, and via constitutionally guaranteed civil rights, or civil liberties, which are manifest as rules and regulations, or statutes, known as civil laws by which citizens associate for the common purposes of "promoting the general welfare, insuring domestic tranquility, and securing the blessings of liberty to ourselves and our posterity."

Being an individual matter, or effort, the defense then of private practice is not properly a Group, Corporate, or Foundation activity but rather that defense is the duty of, the responbility of the individual physician through education in those matters of civil law under which he exercises his license.

In the present cost-conscious third-party atmosphere in which he practices, it is mandatory that the physician be thoroughly informed legally so that he can deal on a one-on-one basis in his civil relationships with those third parties. Physicians have only one thing that third parties want, need, and do not have. That is the knowledge of the art and science of medicine which is manifest by degree and license. Third parties need that license for political-economic reasons and they will try by any means to obtain use of that license. Only the *individual physician, whose license they are after can defend against the various strategies used to get that license.* Only by the preservation of his civil rights, i.e. the security of his license, can the physician retain the freedom necessary to abide by his Code of Ethics.

"Group," "Corporate," and "Foundation" are euphemisms for "Unionism." There are only two reasons for union activity.

1. For employees whose income is dependent on a single source to exert group pressure on that source so as to control that income.

2. For persons who have lost their individual civil rights to act
   as a group to regain those civil rights.

If these latter persons allow themselves to be pulled into the
second category, then they will fall into the first category, the
position of bargaining for their services. *This must not happen in
medicine.* The intelligence that allows that to happen in the first
place cannot ever regain that which it forfeited, i.e., the freedom
of private practice.

Physicians do not fit into the first category because they are
not exployees. They need not fit into the second category but
they are being pulled unwittingly into that category. Physicians
need only to learn how to protect their license, how to prevent
the loss of their civil rights, how to use the *existing legal system*
to prevent that loss. *The legal system is readily available at little
or no cost if used properly.* Only if physicians fail to do this will
they then need Union-type efforts, which, in addition to adding
to social turmoil, can never be successful at bargaining to regain
that which has been forfeited.

So many things go on right under the physician's nose, that
are the demise of private practice, not because they are vio-
lations of his civil rights but because those civil rights are
forfeited by his failure to claim them. Forfeit is no legal violation.

The *only legitimate function of a foundation, or other similar
organization, is to educate physicians in matters mentioned
above.* The TMF does not have this as a purpose.

If thousands of physicians forfeit their civil rights, we have
socialized medicine.

If thousands of physicians, individually, in their private practices, learn how, when, and where to defend their civil rights,
we will *not* have socialized medicine.

The Texas Medical Foundation is off track and by so being
is a greater threat to private practice than government. Government is recognized as an enemy, while the TMF is a Trojan
horse, unrecognized erosion from within.

AMA VS. HEW

Dear Doctor:

Judge Hoffman's decision to grant a temporary injunction against HEW in *AMA et. al. versus HEW* was, in general, a good decision but it contains a most significant and dangerous error.

To review some of his reasoning—on page 9 paragraph 5, Judge Hoffman reiterates a statement by HEW that the consequences of failure to have the "review and certification" is *not* that *the patient* cannot be admitted but only that HEW will not pay the bill. This, of course, is of legal concern only to the hospital and the patient. No physician legal interest is at issue on that point.

It is interesting to note on the same page in paragraphs 6 and 7 that the physician plaintiffs state that these review requirements would cause them not to recommend admission of some patients thus *allowing* third parties to interfere with their medical decisions and in so doing violate Section VI of the Code of Ethics. This also forms the foundation for Judge Hoffman's erroneous opinion to be touched on later.

On page 11 paragraph 4, the judge states that "the review is designed to keep patients out of the hospital and cannot be in the best interests of the patients." He at this point, as above, is not yet giving his opinion but only reiterating points made by defendants and/or plaintiffs and in so doing indicating that these factors will have weight in his opinion. Again, as above, this last quotation is of legal interest only to the patient.

To this point, the judge recognizes that the purpose of the review is twofold: (1) To help determine where the patient will receive the medical treatment he has requested and in so doing (2) determine whether HEW pays for it in the hospital or the patient pays at home. Both issues are of legal interest only to hospitals and patients. Still no justiciable interest for the physician.

It must be recognized before proceeding further that physicians only recommend *where* medical care should be provided. *Where* the patient receives that care is subject to the patient's authority. The doctor's license does not include the legal authority (right) to *dictate* where that care will be given.

Economic factors or arrangements which influence the patient's decision to be hospitalized or remain at home are of *no legal interest* to the physician. In case of hospitalization, the physician's right to exercise his license does not begin until *after* the patient has been admitted. The *doctor's* right therefore is *not contingent on any factors which influence* the patient's decision to be admitted. The doctor's right is the right to make recommendations, i.e., he is licensed to make recommendations, and this right, or this license, is not in fact contingent at any time on where the patient elects to receive recommended care. If the patient chooses to leave the hospital because of third-party terms to which he is contractually bound, the doctor has the free choice of either continuing treatment or withdrawing from the case. He is in violation of Section VI if he continues treatment under conditions contrary to his judgment.

Therefore, the judge is in *error* on page 12 paragraph 4 when he took the bait previously mentioned and stated that "the regulations interfere with a physician's right to practice medicine . . . to . . . a substantial degree . . . " and on that basis gives the AMA/physicians a justiciable interest in this matter, i.e., a legitimate legal reason for filing the suit. To reiterate, that right is not contingent on any factors which influence the patient's decision to be admitted or to remain there until dismissal is recommended by his physician. For a physician to *allow* those factors to *influence his recommendations* is not a violation of that physician's rights but *is a violation by that physician* of Section VI of the Code of Ethics.

This reasoning combined with paragraph 3 page 9 leaves the AMA with no justiciable interest in this matter. The AMA expended funds for defense of legal rights of non-members (patients) and in so doing may have endangered its tax-exempt status, especially in view of the fact that, to my knowledge, it is not empowered by its Constitution and By-Law to defend even its members' civil rights.

The defense of patient's rights is admirable but is the duty of those patients and government. It is good and legally correct for Judge Hoffman to grant a temporary injunction *for the patients* on these issues. A permanent injunction is certainly warranted. Should he do so, it would in essence be a recognition of certain legal principles which are matters of basic law of contract, some of which have been included in court decisions elsewhere. Some of these are:

1. Medicare is a contractual relationship not involving doctors.
2. Its purpose is to pay for health care.
3. By voluntarily assuming that capacity, government is not legally empowered to influence when, where nor how such care is given.
4. In other words, the patient remains free to take his doctor's advice as he sees fit.
5. By agreeing to pay for that care, government cannot legally assume any authority over the doctor.
6. This does not preclude the possibility that the doctor may forfeit certain of his rights through ignorance.
7. No physician has to participate in these programs.
8. No act of a physician in his non-participation role, and either arbitrarily or otherwise can void the government's legal duty to pay for that care, a duty for which it voluntarily contracted under the existing law of contract.

CONCLUSION I:

Physicians have no justiciable interest in these programs in which they are not contractually concerned and which require nothing of them, but they must understand their legal relationship to these programs lest they forfeit certain civil rights by performing certain tasks under the impression they have a legal duty to do so.

CONCLUSION II:

The inexpensive way to settle this matter and others similar is for physicians not to do those things *requested* by government and thereby *force* the hospitals who *are* contractually related and who *would be* the *injured party* to sue HEW for breach of contract with the same net result but at *no cost* to physicians. The AMA expended its funds protecting the legal rights of patients and hospitals *who as contractual partners* with HEW are the only ones with a justiciable interest, and who should have and could have been forced to challenge these issues at their own expense. This holds true for all Utilization-Recertification-PSRO, etc. as is evident in the wording of the Medicare program.

The point in being somewhat critical of the AMA and Judge Hoffman is that if these two parties cannot clarify the legal relationship of all parties concerned, organized medicine did not learn anything from this encounter and will continue to be in trouble as HEW finds ways to circumvent decisions not based on true legal principle.

The fact that AMA/physicians are not a party to this Medicare contractual relationship should have been sufficient reason for the judge to declare the AMA as not having a justiciable interest but would not have changed his opinion since the patients were co-plaintiffs.

A major goal is to get physicians to understand the two basic steps of non-participation:

1. Don't do it yourself.
2. Don't allow your license which is manifest by your History, Physical, Progress Notes, Operative Note, and Discharge Summary to be used for those purposes.
3. If you do allow these written manifestations of your license to be used for purposes of Utilization Review and PSRO, require a paid-in-advance fee.

Yours sincerely,
BEN B. WHITE, M.D.

WEAPON OF CHOICE

Dear Doctor,

Prior to Medicare, the fight to prevent socialized medicine was political, i.e., a fight to block undesirable Congressional legislation. With Medicare, the political battle was lost as the undesirable legislation became a fact. With this legislation, the political perimeter which had protected private practice was penetrated by law. The war continues, but now rages within the compound of "private practice." Since private practice is "individual physicians" exercising individual rights under the civil laws of this nation, the battle has become individual hand-to-hand combat at the office-hospital level. But physicians are in disarray; the individual physician is confused. Neither he nor his leaders understand the nature of the present engagement. They continue to look towards the fallen political perimeter for protection not realizing that this perimeter has collapsed, not realizing that a new strategy, a new weapon, must be used, not realizing that the weapon of choice is at hand. It is useless to continue to depend on and try to strengthen the old political perimeter of organized medicine or to hope for success through the new political perimeter called PAC (Political Action Committee). The weapon at hand, the weapon of choice is not political, it is law, the same law under which the physician exercises his license. Only he can use it; a political perimeter cannot. Each physician must learn what the law of the land really is in respect to his civil rights as a private citizen and he must apply that law. If enough physicians will use the law in this hand-to-hand individual combat situation, private practice will survive. Otherwise it will be overrun; it will perish.

There are two areas in which the private practitioner's individual civil rights are under attack as a result of programs such as Medicare. If the physician loses in either area, it is by forfeit and it is this loss which places his fees and his license under third-party control and is called socialized medicine.

Socialized medicine is:

1. Control of physician's fee by government and
2. Control over the exercise of his medical opinions and decisions, i.e., his license.

The first is occurring as a result of the physician's ignorance of his rights under the law of assignment. The second is occurring in the hospital as a result of the physician's ignorance of the law concerning Utilization Review and PSRO.

Socialized medicine can be prevented by:

1. The proper method of taking assignment and
2. The following amendment to each hospital staff by-law. "No staff member shall be required to submit his records (History, Physical, Progress Notes, Operative Report, or Discharge Summary) to review for the purpose of securing payment of a hospital bill by third parties. The staff shall consider the attending physician's recommendation for admission and dismissal as equivalent to that Ultilization Review and determination of medical necessity which government requires as a condition for payment of the hospital bill. Should government require additional information not available to it from the physician's records, that information must be obtained under separate arrangements."

These two steps are the positive exercise of legal rights under a system of law designed to prevent socialized medicine, a system of law that will not fail if properly used.

This should not be construed as advocating assignment as a routine. In general, the best policy is direct billing, but where circumstances dictate that assignment should be taken, do so in a manner which protects your rights, i.e. your independence (see "Assignments: How to/How Not to").

Sincerely yours,
BEN B. WHITE, M.D.

Part III

Tort Law
vs.
Progress

11
The Jury

The confused, emotional, and seemingly insoluble malpractice issue has become a threat to social stability both as an inflationary pressure on medical economics and a threat to access to professional care. The fact that the controversy continues indicates that the issue has not had proper diagnosis and is being treated only on a symptomatic basis. Such symptomatic treatment will not produce a satisfactory solution but will result only in different undesirable socio-economic manifestations which in the long run will continue to be detrimental to domestic tranquility and liberty.

The problem has multiple facets. It has raised multiple questions in the minds of practitioners, questions which physicians feel do not have answers within the field called Medicine. Some of these questions are:

1. What is the problem which has caused the judiciary to burden the physician with the duty of educating his patients in matters of medicine and surgery under the euphemism "informed consent" when practitioners know that only those trained in medicine can attain truly informed consent while at the same time these uneducated, uninformed people will form the jury to judge his competence should that competence become a legal issue?

2. What is the problem which has produced such an adverse economic environment as to force one to raise his prices contrary to his free-will desire?

3. What is the problem which causes one trained and licensed to be deprived of his right to exercise his license as has happened to many?
4. What is the problem which causes an injured patient to be compensated only if an untrained jury finds negligence but receives nothing if no negligence is found?
5. What is the problem which, *in essence,* places on the physician the duty of guaranteeing that none of his acts as a physician will cause injury by holding him guilty of negligence if injury does occur and is contrary to the intent of the renowned Judge Holmes' expression that "To hold that one must guarantee all against all his acts would be a cruel and unjust burden on all society"—meaning inflation, overcrowded court-dockets, eventual loss of a desirable service, and social stagnation?
6. What is the problem which is converting the cooperative, friendly, very personal, and mutually beneficial doctor-patient relationships into a business adversary relationship tinged with fear, distrust, and even hostility and destructive to the best interests of both parties, society in general and contrary to Section VI of the Physicians' Code of Ethics?
7. What is the problem which has forced 200,000 physicians to carry the economic burden of protecting 200,000,000 against risk of injury?

To the present, most efforts to solve the problem have dealt only with various means of paying for the problem through new legislation which in some manner limits the civil rights of either the lawyer, the patient, or the physician. This is not acceptable. A solution which will establish fault and just compensation without compromising the civil rights of either party must be found.

There seems to be two major areas which are the primary sources of confusion in the issue. These are:

1. Determination of fault.
2. Compensation for damages.

In the first, the issue which appears to be the source of basic disagreement but has not been isolated and identified as such is "Should fault be determined by trained physicians or an untrained jury?" This issue has led to the recognition by many that some type of arbitration panel, review board or screening panel is needed so that those who are trained and qualified to decide the issue may in some manner strongly influence the outcome. But because no one is willing to do away with our long established jury system, such arbitration or screening cannot be legally binding. Here is an area of confusion or conflict, a recognition of a need but apparently no legal way to fit the need into the existing and desirable legal structure.

This problem stems from failure of the judicial-legislative processes to adjust Tort law to the educational-communications-transportation-population changes called "progress" which have resulted in greatly increased and more complicated social contacts and therefore greatly increased chance of injury as the result of one's association and participation in society. In other words, the law which has allowed progress has not adjusted to that progress and if it does not adjust will exert an anchoring effect on progress. (It was reasonable to say negligence when a T-Model doing 30 mph ran into the rear of another on a dirt road fifty years ago with no other traffic in sight; but is it reasonable to use the same terminology for a Houston freeway at 7:30 A.M. rather than just use the word "accident"?)

Jury trial is a two-hundred-year-old institution in this country. That statement has some significance in that two hundred years ago, the citizens of this country, agrarian orientated, were more or less equally educated and were more or less each other's peer. But progress has produced markedly different degrees of learning and skill so that there are numerous areas in which certain persons are highly trained and skilled while the great majority of the citizenry is ignorant of this training and its application. Yet those highly trained individuals, in the application of their training, are to be judged by randomly selected and untrained citizens. *This is not reasonable.* It is not reasonable to hold that any professional in the exercise of his license must practice according to the standards of a "reasonable and prudent man of similar professional standing" and then deny him the right to have his practice judged by those same reasonable and prudent men but rather be judged by men who by virtue of ignorance cannot possibly reach reasonable and prudent decisions but can only reach decisions based on emotion and individual unrelated experience influenced by oratory and rhetoric. What can be more illogical than having untrained men decide which expert is right?

A comparable situation would be to have a criminal code by which all are to abide but then not allow one on trial for violation of that code to be judged by that code.

This is not to imply that physicians are not to be subject to some degree of policing. But quality of medical care is not determined by legislation nor judicial decree nor can it be improved by economic and personal harassment of those trained and licensed to provide it. Quality is determined by the intelligence, ability, motivation and training plus continued practice and continuing education of those licensed to provide that care together with the intelligence, confidence and capability of the recipient of that care. As an intangible, quality is not subject to written standards as in civil and criminal law and must therefore be judged by the intangible standard of a "Reasonal and Prudent Man" of similar training. It was the recognition that civil and criminal statutes cannot adequately protect or police the public interest in this intangible area that caused practitioners to adopt the Code of Ethics to accomplish that protective function. It is an inescapabe conclusion that only physicians can properly police and judge the acts of physicians in the exercise of their license.

The definition of jury seemingly supports this thesis. The definitions use the words "competent" or "qualified" for the members. A legal clarification of those terms is indicated. Are just "physically fit" and "sane" to be adequate, or should they mean "of similar acquired knowledge and skill" also?

Two hundred years ago or even a hundred years ago, most people provided for most of their needs themselves and seldom *requested* services, especially technical services, of others. Most services which are now available did not exist then. Another area of possible judicial deficiency is therefore raised by the question, "Why has Tort law not adjusted to this progress by establishing different standards of care for injury as the result of unrequested acts versus injury from requested services?" The resolution of this should produce the same result as would meaningful definitions of "qualified" or "competent" with regard to jurors. In other words, the standard of care for injuries from requested services would be that of a "Reasonable and Prudent Man" as determined by a qualified jury rather than an unqualified jury.

Is our legal system to be so rigid, so inflexible, that it cannot keep in step with the society, the progress for which the legal system is responsible, and by such obstinance be the cause of social instability, stagnation, and eventual deterioration to an archaic or medieval society and system of government presently and euphemistically referred to as "socialistic," or is it to be intelligently and analytically responsive to the social pressures caused by progress and thereby continue its role of "insuring domestic tranquility, promoting the general welfare and securing the blessing of liberty to ourselves and our posterity"?

12
Negligence and Domestic Tranquility

The second area of concern, that of compensation for injury, is even more complicated.

The malpractice issue is a reflection of, and hopefully will focus attention on a serious, a potentially fatal illness, afflicting our society, an illness which is eroding our peaceful cooperative association environment and is largely responsible for the symptoms called "deterioration of the national moral fiber." This is frequently expressed as "people are not the same anymore; they don't care, etc." This illness, if unchecked, will be fatal to the social atmosphere which is a national spirit of concern and respect for each individual's safety, rights, and property, or in other words it will be fatal for those conditions which are "domestic tranquility."

This affliction, this illness, is gradually, as the result of progress, causing more and more social friction, instability, stagnation and even regression while overcrowding the courts as it turns people into adversaries. It is destroying the sense of national unity and providing a foundation for dictatorial government so subtly that the majority are unaware of its presence. It does so by feeding on that basic weakness of human nature called "greed."

Many people are aware of the symptoms of this national disintegration but are unable to identify the culprit. The culprit is the Tort law concept of negligence. The negligence concept is an old, well-established legal doctrine which may have served a useful purpose but has outlived its usefulness and may now be an albatross. As a concept which allows one to hold others responsible for injury which occurs to his person or property as a result of his association and participation in society rather than being responsible for his own physical and economic security, it tends to destroy individual responsibility. Its continued implementation by the courts conditions the people to accept the development of a dictatorial government in that the people become more conditioned to depend on others for their tangible physical and economic security and to accept the intangible losses of liberty which accrue as authoritarian government attempts to meet the tangible desires.

The concept of negligence must be reevaluated if our national unity is to be restored and our national security preserved, because the disease it causes spreads to and destroys other areas of the national structure as the citizens, with judicial support, become more willing to promote their own interests (greed) at the expense of others. In so doing, concern for the safety and rights of others is lost. The national character then becomes not only unwilling to defend the person, rights, and property of others as manifest by a passive, unconcerned, insecure society, and even a weakened military, but also more willing to damage or destroy the person, property, and rights of others as manifest by rising crime and greatly increased civil suits. The present trend hailed by members of the profession is to counter-sue for frivolous unjustified suits. It will be exceedingly unfortunate if this proves to be one of the solutions to the problem because this will only serve to widen the chasm between medicine and the public by causing them to be virtual adversaries thus aiding in the destruction of domestic tranquility.

The concept of negligence is destruction from within, working favorably for those who are anxious for the demise of this great nation, as it effectively implements the theory of "divide and conquer."

The entire concept of social injury is in critical need of study to find a free enterprise means by which one can voluntarily protect himself from injury as a result of his associations in this more densely populated and sophisticated society and in a manner which will neutralize those latent forces which threaten domestic tranquility.

Are we to succumb to this disease or do we diagnose, treat, and continue to progress because of domestic tranquility, which *is* concern and respect for and willingness to protect the person, property and rights of others and is called a "strong national moral fiber"?

This nation is comparable to a 200,000,000-man football team in a world football conference. What happens to its position in that conference if the rules of the game remain unchanged but the rules which govern the individual team members encourages those members to become adversaries with their time spent in litigation for personal gain rather than on the practice field? What happens when those rules cause team friction and dissent rather than a spirit of mutual cooperation and concern for each other's safety and well being, a spirit which is domestic tranquility and which encourages the effort which secures for us first place, which is the "blessing of liberty"? What happens? The answer is obvious, we develop internal strife, progress ceases, and freedom is lost. We become a last-place team.

13
Fiction vs. Reality

The general discontent evident in many facets of society is diametrically opposed to domestic tranquility and should be sufficient warning to those who are responsible for domestic tranquility that basic defects exist in our rules of association.

The conduct of society as a whole depends on the conduct of the individual members. The conduct of an individual becomes a matter of legal or judicial consideration when that conduct injures someone else. At this level of law, the conduct of the individual is judged according to the standard of a "Reasonable and Prudent Man" when the injury concerned was not intentional and not a result of violation of criminal statutes.

The law has considerable difficulty defining the "Reasonable and Prudent Man." It defines him, more or less, as a "perfect man," one who in any given situation would not have reacted in such a manner as to cause the injury that did occur. If one does not meet this standard of perfection then he is said to be negligent if his imperfection causes injury, and he is liable for damages which accrue.

Such a perfect man is of course an impossibility. It is understandable therefore when one reads in these law books that this concept is a figment of the imagination, a fiction created to solve a problem which apparently has no other solution. This just means that the law has not yet discovered a satisfactory method of compensating for social injury founded on the logical and factual premise that man is not perfect. Unfortunately, neither the courts nor the legislatures have seen fit to cause any research in this direction.

Because man and his associations are not fiction, this fictional concept would appear to be on shaky grounds. It does indeed arouse a strong suspicion that it is a cause of domestic friction rather than domestic tranquility.

The legal concept of a "Reasonable and Prudent Man" becomes operative *after* an injury has occurred as the result of an act or failure to act by an imperfect person. Because this concept relieves an individual of the responsibility for his own safety and security in his associations by placing that responsibility on others, it establishes an adversary atmosphere for all rather than that inherently cooperative atmosphere of mutual respect called domestic tranquility. This adversary atmosphere is characterized by distrust, discontent and lack of concern for the safety and property rights of others as manifest by rising crime, overcrowded courts and social stagnation as untold manhours are spent in socially unproductive litigation and preparation for litigation.

It's time to abandon the back door, fictional concept of negligence with the "Reasonable and Prudent Man" as a retrospective standard of care. It's time we accept ourselves as ordinary people and provide a governing environment in which ordinary people can exert their liberty with a feeling of tranquility. It's time to use common sense as the standard of care and remove the divisive atmosphere which results when one is allowed to hold others financially responsible for any real and/or imaginary troubles which befall him as a result of his associations. It's time to deal with society as individuals who, in general, inherently feel responsible for their own safety and security, individuals who will exercise that responsibility if given the proper legislative-judicial atmosphere in which to do so. It's time to deal with society head-on, as a reality, made up of people who are not infallable, people who are not constantly alert, people who do not have crystal balls, people who will make mistakes in judgment, people who will cause injury to others, injury which is neither intentional or criminal, injury therefore which by all standards of reason should be called accidental.

Why take forever no-faulting the different areas of human association with complex legislation as those areas become more involved in litigation rather than recognizing and correcting a basic fault?

It is proposed that consideration be given to Social Accident Insurance. It would compensate for actual damages but remove from the field of litigation those intangibles such as pain, suffering, and loss of conjugal rights, etc., which, as life itself, are not subject to reasonable monetary evaluation and are the cause of severely inflated awards. If those intangibles are to be given monetary value, then, for economic ballast, that valuation must be done by the individual concerned who must be able to pay the cost of protecting whatever value he places on his life, comfort, conjugal rights, etc.

Under this concept, Mr. Average American becomes the logical, nonfictional reasonable and prudent man who, recognizing the fallibility of his fellowman, uses this method to protect his interests by purchasing coverage as he desires. Anyone who fails to avail himself of this protection would be presumed to consider his fellow man to be perfect and not capable of causing injury. Such an individual would be deemed not reasonable and prudent and therefore not deserving of consideration by the judicial system anymore than one who is aware of the uncertainty of time of death is deserving to have his heirs awarded if he fails to carry life insurance.

This is the front door approach, it is the reasonable and prudent approach, it is economically sound, it will relieve the present burden on the judicial system by retaining potential litigants in their normal productive capacities in society as it replaces the divisive adversary atmosphere with the atmosphere of mutual respect, cooperation, individual responsibility and called domestic tranquility.

It is not fiction; it is reality.

14
A Change of Horses

When pressures, in the form of inflated cost of and/or lack of availability of a service essential to the national welfare, occur in a free enterprise society to the extent that governmental intervention, with its accompanying loss of civil rights, is encouraged, without public dissent and even with public approval, those pressures are but the result of failure of government to perform its duty of providing a proper legislative and judicial atmosphere in which people do for themselves. People doing for themselves is the free enterprise system. When government undertakes to do for people, it can do no more than that which the people would have done for themselves under the proper legislative and judicial environment and without loss of those rights which invariably occur with governmental intervention.

There is an eminent crisis in the field of services called the Practice of Medicine. The public is faced with the real danger of rapidly rising cost of medical care and/or severely restricted availability of that service.

Present efforts of the various states to resolve the problem cannot be successful in that these efforts cannot resolve the problem without sacrifice of certain civil rights of the parties concerned. *Such sacrifice is not acceptable.* These efforts deal with the problem *after* an event has occurred which leads to the establishment of a lawyer-patient relationship. Such relationships are a manifestation of social friction and instability rather than social tranquility. These efforts will not be beneficial to the national interest because the lawyer-patient relationship injects many intangible factors which cannot be equitably related to the tangible economic system and will therefore continue to cause severe abuse of the economic system while exerting no effort to remove divisive forces.

The development of a lawyer-patient relationship must therefore be circumvented in order to secure domestic tranquility. It must be circumvented by a legitimate means which is more acceptable to the public, a method which will satisfactorily compensate for actual injury with a minimum of effort compared to the present method of litigation, a method which will allow the injured party to continue in the care of his personal physician without impairment of that relationship, a method which will prevent the necessity of violating the lawyer's civil rights by *mandatory* limitations on contingency fees and the patient's civil rights by *mandatory* limitations on awards and/or mandatory arbitration while still allowing compensations regardless of fault.

One of the basic differences between a free enterprise system and the socialistic systems is the insurance industry. The ultimate goal of the free enterprise system is to preserve liberty or freedom from restraints because we, as a society, have learned that the greatest progress is possible in an environment of freedom. The insurance concept is a natural economic adaptation to this thesis. As a free will development, it helps to provide the individual with the security which allows him to exercise the freedom necessary to cause progress. The insurance concept allows anyone, by virtue of a small premium, to protect himself against the statistical possibility of injury either physical or economic which could destroy his economic security and therefore his independence.

In the field of malpractice, the insurance concept has been misapplied with the result that 200,000 physicians have become responsible for protecting two hundred million people against risk of injury as a result of requested medical care.

This can be corrected by offering to the people a means whereby they can voluntarily protect themselves against unforeseen injury as a result of requested medical care, a method which will compensate equitably, more rapidly, without creating hostility and divisiveness, without unjust enrichment of uninjured parties, and without damaging the economy related to the service nor the availability of that service.

It is proposed that Medical Accident insurance be offered to the public. This would, of course, be available before the fact. In these contracts which would cost approximately $50 per year per family, many of the more common causes of litigation would be specified and other injuries would be subject to voluntarily binding arbitration by qualified persons. The contract would allow for compensation either by the insurance mechanism or litigation *but not both*. Since present procedure produces prolonged litigation and a low percentage of judgments in favor of the patient with an ultimate recovery of only about 20 percent of the settlement or judgment, it is anticipated that the public would rather take a "bird in hand" than the rather remote possibility of "four in the bush" especially since the four in the bush are acquired only with great difficulty and risk, and, after caught, melt into one, i.e. a $100,000 judgment or settlement will leave the patient with approximately $20,000.

If Medical Accident insurance is offered to the public and achieves public acceptance, it will be another demonstration of the great importance of the insurance industry as a major factor in a free enterprise economy.

It must be recognized on the medical and public front that quality of medical care, i.e. freedom from injury as a result of medical care, cannot be improved by assault on the profession. Quality of care is a product of training, ability, practice and many more intangibles. It can be maintained and improved only by continuing practice and continuing education under conditions conducive to learning and motivation of the practitioner.

This approach would be of benefit to the public interest because it would solve the problem without additional legislation to complicate our relationships and without infringement on individual civil rights.

CONCLUSION

The difference between human relations *now* and a hundred years ago is progress. Were it not for progress, Tort law could adjudicate injury issues as well now as then. Progress, however, *is* more complicated relationships such as the practice of medicine, relationships which are the result of application of special acquired knowledge and skills not available a century ago. Homo sapiens, as a very fallible creature, with neither microscopic nor X-ray vision, ESP, nor crystal ball—not omnipotent—can, in the application of this knowledge and skill, produce unexpected and unintentional injury. He has failed to establish a legal mechanism which will equitably compensate for injury due to inherent human imperfection in the application of his skill. Under the condition of imperfection, his government holds him to perfection as a standard of care under the euphemistic, nebulous, indefinable phrase "a Reasonable and Prudent Man." This retrospective standard of care requires those who qualify themselves to provide progress to be the sole responsible party for all adverse results of that progress. That is bad policy, poor government. Those who benefit from progress must also share in its risks if society is to have progress. To hold otherwise is a sure way to produce social stagnation and regression, a return to the dark ages of feudalism or socialism, as those with the ability not only lose their motivation to render their service but become financially unable to do so.

The most *acceptable* solution to the malpractice problem is to distribute the risk through society as Medical Accident Insurance. Whatever needs to be done to accomplish that must be done.

The question "What is medical accident?" was asked by the President's Commission, but it failed to answer the question. Statistics show that of all injury cases filed less than 5 percent are found against the doctor, i.e. were the result of negligence.

The rest of these injuries were medical accidental injuries, injuries against which the public at present has no mechanism available to protect itself except to sue and then 95 percent unsuccessfully.

An alternative to the establishment of the time-consuming, hostile, lawyer-client-defendant relationship with its high cost, unlimited damages, and contingency fees, must be provided . . . an alternative by which the public also assumes a degree of risk for the benefits of progress. This alternative is Medical Accident Insurance. It would give the public the choice of collecting for injury through the insurance channel or through action at Tort, but not both.

To reiterate, whatever needs to be done to implement this concept, must be done.

Part IV

The Physician's Non-Medical Responsibility

15
Ethics and Law

Policing of human associations is a long recognized prerequisite for a safe and progressive association. This policing is accomplished by those two broad categories called Civil and Criminal law. The desire for progress caused the creation of centers of higher learning which produce individuals with knowledge and skill the remainder of society does not have and therefor does not know when that knowledge and skill is being properly applied. Society is therefore at the mercy of those so trained who are unscrupulous. The degree of progress which society obtains from these specially trained individuals depends on whether the individual remains abreast of the progress in his field which, as the original training, is subject only to his volition. Organized medicine has long recognized the inability of civil and criminal statutes to protect the public interest in the specialized field called Medicine so it adopted the burden of protecting the public interest as an ethical duty. The public trust is of necessity placed in the Code of Ethics but to the present time, organized medicine has not recognized that its ethical duty extends to requiring that the physician keep abreast of current knowledge in his field of practice.

It is therefore recommended that the AMA add to its Code of Ethics a section which provides that "a physician shall remain abreast of current developments in his field of practice."

CONSTITUTIONAL GUARANTEES

This nation was established as a result of our forefathers' desire to live in an atmosphere free of unreasonable governmen-

tal restraint. They manifest their desire by declaring their independence, establishing their authority to do so by use of military
power, and then transferring the authority for the desired liberty
from military power to writing. That Constitution has endured
as the authority by which to be governed in such a manner as to
guarantee liberty, or absence of restraint, for present and future
generations. We are the posterity then mentioned, the fortunate
beneficiaries of their efforts. As practitioners of medicine, we are
faced with threats to that freedom, the freedom to exercise our
license according to training, to be free of unreasonable restraints. As a people, our liberty again is in jeopardy. What
course of action do we take?

Physicians, by virtue of training, are solely responsible for the
quality of medical care the public receives. *We must remain
free of governmental restraints if quality of care is to be maintained at a high level. We have an ethical duty not to allow
third-party interests, i.e., economic restraints, to result in economizing medical care. We have an ethical duty to remain free.
The Constitution provides for that freedom as a legal right. It
also provides the mechanics by which to have freedom without
need for either rebellion, unionization, or use of the force to
which our forefathers had to resort.*

The Constitution is the substitute for that force.

Physicians must realize that the socialization process is the
loss of their freedom. It is the loss of physician civil rights. But
so long as we have the Constitution, that loss is a loss by forfeit.
Without the realization of the nature of the war being waged
against them, physicians will never understand how to fight it,
and without that understanding they cannot possibly win it.

In the present governing atmosphere which threatens our
freedom, physicans must learn to assert, to claim, their guaranteed rights, their liberty. Freedom is there, in the Constitution,
just for the taking.

Existing organizations have not yet recognized the mechanics
of the socialization process. These organizations continue to use
the weapon of politics in a battle that is being waged on the
legal front. The AMA has in the past fought the political battle

well. Through politics it *prevented* Murray-Wagner-Dingle, King-Anderson, Kerr-Mills, etc.: but in 1966, with Medicare, *the political phase of the war to prevent federal control was lost. If we continue to fight a legal war with a weapon of politics, we are doomed to failure.* We must adopt a different approach, a new weapon; we must fight law with law. We need not necessarily engage in litigation but only understand what really is the law of the land, what our civil rights are in respect to third parties so that the war can be won at minimal expense in the course of the normal conduct of the practice of medicine. Physicians must learn something of basic constitutional law, basic contract law, basic assignment law, those basic laws under which they now conduct their practices, but about which they are so oblivious. This knowledge will enable them individually to use that law to deal with third parties on a one-on-one basis and stop having to depend on organizations for the preservation of their freedom.

No one but the individual whose right is at issue has the authority to preserve it; organizations cannot prevent socialization, only individual physicians can.

Two basic principles must be recognized:

1. The designation "M.D." does not alter one's relationship with the civil statutes which govern this nation. Your civil rights are unchanged. You have no greater authority over others nor do others have any greater authority over you. You have voluntarily assumed the single additional legal duty of providing medical care and advice with reasonable care and skill, nothing else can be *required* of you. It may be requested of you, yes, but not required. It is no legal violation for you, through ignorance, to forfeit your civil rights.
2. Socialism is not a self-propelled entity which can go forward of its own legal power. It is an ever-present evil which is sucked into the vacuum created when free men retreat before the political pressure of the utopian circle by failure to use the legal system designed for the purpose of preventing that type of government.

If enough physicians develop an understanding that will enable them to adopt and use the folowing physicians' Declaration of Independence, knowing the Constitution stands behind it, we will not have Socialized Medicine. We must act now. Will posterity be fortunate? Will they benefit from our efforts? Will they benefit from our Declaration?

PHYSICIAN'S DECLARATION OF INDEPENDENCE

We, the physicians of the USA, hold to the belief of our forefathers that the ultimate mortal goal for which all people yearn is liberty with justice for all.

We desire to retain this liberty in order to provide quality medical care for which we alone are trained and for which we hold ourselves solely responsible.

We intend to exercise whatever legal rights are necessary to preserve that liberty.

We hereby declare that we recognize that our acquired knowledge neither grants us greater nor deprives us of any of the civil rights bestowed on all citizens of this country. We further recognize that the only additional legal duty bestowed on us by virtue of our acquired knowledge is the duty to dispense medical advice and care with reasonable care.

We therefore *declare* that we will perform acts requested by third parties *only at our discretion and if so at all only as either recommendations to those third parties or their agents or under such contractual terms as will protect our civil liberties thereby fulfilling both the ethical obligation of remaining free of nonmedical influence when rendering medical care and the moral obligation of preserving liberty for ourselves and our posterity.*

16
Recommendations to AMA

1. Furnish all present and future physicians with a copy of this book, not that everything in it is correct, but to give them a different perspective and a new hope.
2. Advise physicians to take assignment when indicated according to the terms recommended herein; and,
3. When assignment is not taken, to give better assurance of payment, provide the patient only with the amount of the bill until it is paid with cash, check, credit card, or promissory note.
4. Charge for additional information requested by third parties.
5. Cease doing Utilization Review.
6. Separate physician's part of hospital record from the remainder.
7. Provide for Liaison Committee only between Hospital Board of Trustees and Medical Staff.
8. AMA establish a Medical Staff Accreditation Committee and ignore JCAH.
9. Recommend to physicians that the Medical Staff alone determines who its members will be.
10. Work towards adoption of "Medical Accident Insurance" concept and a national re-evaluation of the tort concept of negligence.
11. Abolish all medical foundations.
12. Membership in local medical society be required as a condition for hospital staff membership.
13. Separate Constitution and By-Law for non-M.D. providers of care.

14. Do not delineate privileges.
15. M.D.'s be licensed for the field of practice concerned after completion of the prescribed course of training.
16. Organize and encourage financial support for an organization to be the individual physician's advocate in matters pertaining to his civil rights insofar as the practice of medicine is concerned.
17. Change Section VII of the Code of Ethics to read "A physician shall remain abreast of current developments and progress in her/his field of practice."
18. Change present Section VII to Section VIII; Section VIII to Section IX, Section IX to X and Section X to XI.
19. Make an in-depth study of the concept of "Insurance" as applied to illness and accident.
20. Require a three-month course in Tort law and Contract law as either a prerequisite for medical school or during senior year of medical school.
21. Adopt the "Physician's Declaration of Independence."

Part V

Thoughts for
Conservatives

17
Conservative Goals

Socialist theory teaches that socialized medicine is the cap-
stone that completes and supports the arch of socialism. The
prevention of socialized medicine therefore is, or should be, a
prime goal of conservatism. This book has placed its major
emphasis on the cause and prevention of socialized medicine.
Hopefully, physicians will respond to this information and other
professionals perhaps will understand that the basic principles
presented apply to them also. The prevention of socialized medicine however, will not relieve the pressure for socialization.
More must be done.

These comments are directed to conservatives in general to
give them a different view of the meaning of conservatism with
the hopes that they will develop a better understanding of their
cause, their goals, and how to achieve them.

Conservatism is a force in politics. It always will be, but the
degree of influence will depend on the degree of understanding
that conservatives have of their cause.

Each election year finds conservatism short in its efforts to
gain the reins of power. This probably is good, at least for the
present, because conservatives apparently do not have a full
understanding of either their principles or the true source of their
political power. They do not seem to know how to exploit their
own strength nor the weakness of their liberal opponents. They
would therefore be unable to transmit their ideas, their principles, to governing authority. The resulting failure as a government would mean the relegation of conservatism to the political
graveyard. The ranges of government would then, for practical

purposes, be open only to liberals, a most unfortunate event for future generations.

During the major political campaigns, hopes are raised high as millions of voters cheer the rhetoric which proclaims the defense of liberty, the intangible freedom, but in the ballot booth, these hopes are dashed as millions of Januses again take up the pursuit of Utopia and cast their vote for tangible comfort.

After each major election, conservatives gather to analyze events, to regroup, to plan new strategy. "How do we continue to be an influence on the governing process?" And they invariably find themselves talking not of intangible principles, but of tangible politics to get back into the mainstream not understanding that the mainstream is the pursuit of Utopia, a pursuit which inevitably leads to totalitarianism. Tangibles are offered as a reward for votes. The conservative who desires to defend the intangible freedom rather than to feed on it finds himself succumbing to political pressure, preying on that which he is dedicated to preserving. The conservatives, the men of principle, under the pressure of politics, weaken, and a little left shift occurs within their ranks. This is the reason Communists so patiently believe in the inevitability of socialism and communism, the socially acceptable terms for modern feudalism. The forces of the vicious circle cause the conservative Republican or Democrat or Independent of today, poorly grounded in the theory and principles of freedom, to be tomorrow's liberal Republican or Democrat; the liberal of today to be tomorrow's Socialist, and the Socialist of today to be tomorrow's Communist. Lack of understanding causes the gradual shift of governments to the left.

The world societies are caught in a great political pump, the increasing tangible, or material accomplishments, produced by a few and attained by a few more, and which far outstrips the average attained level of comfort on the one hand, and the desire of the masses for that greater comfort on the other hand. The socializing forces are those which try too quickly to close the gap, to pull or push all to the peak without regard for preparation, for ability, for liberty, only to have them slide off later while the Conservative may never get them to the peak because of inability to properly equip, to properly prepare society to go to the peak under its own power with liberty so that the high ground can be held for all posterity once it is attained. Conservative and Liberal have the same goal, a society with maximum prosperity and tranquility, but Conservatives concentrate more on preserving the inherently desired liberty while Liberals concentrate on attaining the inherently desired material goals. Neither appreciates fully the existence of, the necessity of satisfying both desires. The great majority of liberals are also conservative (or perhaps that should be "the great majority of conservatives are also liberal"). The minority of those who call themselves liberal are really socialistic (or should that be "the minority of those who call themselves conservative are really right-wingers")? The problem with socialism is that it revokes the freedom which is necessary to prevent its progression to communism (or perhaps that should be "the problem with right-wing extremism is that it revokes the freedom which is necessary to prevent its progression to fascism"). Fear of that progression is the reason conservatives are so anti-liberal, anti-socialist (or should that be "fear of that progression is the reason liberals are so anti-conservative, anti-rightist")? In any event, both sides have failed. Neither appreciates fully either the reason for its stance or the commonality of goals. This lack of understanding, this failure, is a major cause of the divisiveness which is manifest by the names "liberal" and "conservative" and is called "politics."

Conservatism's failure is the failure to recognize the two inherent drives, the two faces, of the voting public, the two basic desires of human nature mentioned in "The Vicious Circle," the desire for the tangible comfort and the desire for the intangible freedom, and to establish symbiosis between these desires and conservatism. It is the failure to recognize that today's conservatism is the politics only of the intangible freedom while Liberalism is the politics of the tangible comfort. It is the failure to recognize that the power of the pressure on Liberal politicians is a measure of the difference between known levels of attainable comfort, or materialistic progress, and the average attained level of materialistic progress. The more affluent are more likely to give more consideration to the intangible freedom and to vote conservative while the underprivileged will vote for the tangible comfort. So it may be said that the power of the pressure on Liberal politicians is inversely proportional to the average level of material achievement which in turn is, in general, proportional to the average level of educational achievement. Conservatism's failure is the failure to recognize that its strength is the intelligence, the understanding of the people and its weakness is their ignorance while ignorance is the strength of Liberalism and wisdom is its weakness. Conservatism's failure is the lack of platforms which would accentuate conservative strength and liberalism's weakness. Such platforms must eventually reduce the political pressure to which liberal politicians must respond and produce governing officials whose understanding would reduce their susceptibility to that political pressure. Such platforms would be readily acceptable to the public as they would be founded primarily on improved educational achievement, understanding for all. Such platforms, by correcting root causes of social adversity, would provide such general security, comfort, domestic tranquility, and freedom as to leave minimal pressure to activate Liberal politicians.

Conservatives must not look just to today, tomorrow, and next year but to the distant future. They must discover the issues which have intangible political strength, i.e., strong public support even though those issues do not cater directly to individual comfort; issues which will obviously produce national and individual comfort and liberty, issues which furnish the ties that bind; issues which change social adversity, social friction, to domestic tranquility.

Conservatives must answer the questions:

1. What is the source of progress?
2. What are the root-causes of social stagnation, regression, friction, welfare, crime, etc., and how can they be corrected?
3. How can we assure the election of governing officials who are not so inclined to respond to selfish political pressure?

The issues which are destructive to domestic tranquility insofar as health care is concerned plus the general destabilizing effect of the tort concept of negligence have been discussed and recommendations made.

The following are recommendations for conservatives to evaluate. Recognize as the equation for successful human association (Intelligence + Freedom) × (Ability + Effort) = Prosperity + Tranquility, an equation which recognizes education, freedom, and effort as being the primary sources of progress.

Public Education:

The ratio between the education received in the public school system and that needed for a productive capacity in society has been greatly altered during the past half century. This preparedness ratio could be greatly improved by lengthening the public school term to fifteen years. This would provide a better trained, more capable, more content future populace with less motivation towards chaos. It would relieve the colleges of the burden of those who shouldn't be there. In the long run, it would reduce the welfare rolls and the crime rate. A further consequence would be a reduction in the number of teen-age marriages and a fewer number of teenagers in the military. The reduction of teen-age marriages would reduce the divorce rate while the reduction of teenagers in the military would produce a greater military stability and happier parents. During these extra three years, courses in child psychology and the *principles of liberty*, the free enterprise system would be required. Graduation from high school would be required as a prerequisite for military service and marriage. Failure to graduate would reduce future welfare or Social Security benefits by fifty percent.

The issue of discipline in schools has resulted in court restrictions on punishment by teachers. A prerequisite for learning is a disciplined atmosphere. Discipline is not provided by teachers. Discipline is within the student. It is his respect for the authority and purpose of the teacher. Parents who desire a disciplined atmosphere so that their children can be educated should arise.

They should sign statements giving the teachers the power of punishment in order to have a disciplined atmosphere. The court restrictions on punishment do not deprive the parents of the right to a disciplined schoolroom but they must exercise that right. Any parents who do not wish their children to be subject to the school's punishment would have their children taught in separate classrooms where discipline would be absent. It is not logical for parents to delegate to the schools the most important part of their child's life, his education, and deny those schools the authority by which to attain a disciplined atmosphere in which to attain that goal.

Marriage:

The family unit, the basic building block of a free society is being destroyed by divorce. Divorce adds to domestic friction as children from broken homes in general provide destabilizing forces on society. Divorce is the result of inadequate preparation for marriage. The use of the word "license" in marriage license is a mockery. It is a permit, but it should be a license to indicate qualification for that undertaking. The requirements for marriage basically are no different in this complex sophisticated society than they were two hundred years ago. In this society, there should be certain qualifications for marriage so that the marriage will be a stabilizing factor in society rather than the reverse. A high school diploma should be required along with a course in basic child psychology. Such requirements would greatly relieve the problem of economic instability which is usually a factor in divorce, improve the overall home atmosphere and thereby improve the quality of life of the couple and the children of those marriages. This would promote domestic tranquility.

Womens Rights:

It is an indisputable law of nature that only females will experience the inequality of suffering the physical pain of perpetuating the human race and being compensated for that suffering by being entitled, by physical design and mental characteristics, to the designation "Mother" to reap the reward of pleasure and responsibility of a unique relationship which is the primary influence on the development of the personality and character which will determine to a large degree the future happiness and success an individual has in his associations as a member of the human race. The laws of nature deny the male that relationship with his offspring but compensate him by providing through physical design and mental characteristics that he be the protector, the guardian of that most beautiful of all relationships, the one to face the dangers of the world, to be the provider of food and shelter, the leader, the authority, the security for the family, in short, the father. If we are to have laws which require that women have the same rights and opportunities in their relationships outside the family, in society, as the men who are by nature deprived of the unique "Mother" status, we should also have laws which recognize these basic laws of nature by requiring mothers to be home with those children to exercise the natural designation of mother while the father is exercising his natural designation during the formative years of the child's life.

Abortion:

God placed his trust for the reproduction of mankind, the perpetuation of mankind in woman with full awareness that the free-will which he also provided may act adversely to that purpose. In his wisdom, he provided the protective instincts of motherhood. Man should not presume to overrule God's wisdom. Where pregnancy occurs, especially as a result of free-will, man should not make laws regarding the continuance of that pregnancy, but leave the matter between God and the individual woman. Man's concern should be limited to deciding, in the interest of the woman's safety, the latest time that she can safely have an abortion if she so decides and to seeing that such abortion is done according to accepted medical standards.

Policemen:

For society to expect a man to become either a superman or a robot by virtue of donning a police uniform is totally unreasonable. A uniform does not change basic humanity, basic desires, basic fears, basic instincts. Officers daily place their lives in jeopardy for our benefit. They are extremely sensitized, by daily experience to the threat of physical harm or death, and they are not immune to injury or fear. The uniform does not relieve them of either the normal desires to be unharmed or to see criminals punished which is supposedly the reason for the risk they take to apprehend and detain.

It is very unfortunate that our judicial system has gradually assumed a posture which does not enforce or apparently even support the efforts of our officers. Police officers are civilian soldiers. What would be the result if soldiers under combat conditions took prisoners only to have their commanders return those prisoners to the enemy to be re-armed, to be faced again on the battlefield? I daresay those soldiers, in the name of personal safety and survival, would cease their efforts to take prisoners. Is that then to be called brutality? We must recognize that other factors influence the occurrence of brutality. If the judicial system would take proper action against those apprehended; if the purpose of the officers' efforts and risks were accomplished, i.e., if justice were dispensed, there would be much less psychic pressure on officers to serve up such justice at the time of arrest. The answer to brutality does not lie in retrospective analysis, even by trained officers, much less untrained review boards. The situation at the time of arrest cannot be reproduced by such boards. The circumstances which provoked the act have been altered considerably. It's like trying to judge whether a lawn needs watering thirty minutes after the sprinkler has been turned on. All the tangible and intangible factors affecting the judgment no longer exist. The answer to brutality lies in good training, excellent physical condition, willingness to use all force necessary, and a demonstration of that willingness, but most of all in justice for the apprehended criminal.

If we ever have a police force made up of namby-pamby-turn-the-other-cheek officers who have been subdued by fear of reprisal for exercising a judgment which is formed from original competence, training, and experience, then we no longer have a police force. The public must learn to accept the perfections and imperfections of those selected and trained in a field of endeavor and when enough incidents occur which dictate that change is in order, those changes should occur at the level of selection, training and command if there is to be unanimity and uniformity. To make issues of isolated events is haphazard, not beneficial, chaotic, and leaves the individual officers in a position of uncertainty and insecurity, both of which are detrimental to the proper function of their duties. We are a society much too quick to jump at the occasional imperfections of our fellow man rather than being extremely grateful for the ninety-eight percent excellent performance that we get from all our areas of association.

Capital Punishment:

A cause of considerable debate and marked differences of opinion, and social friction, is the issue of capital punishment. No one denies that criminals should be punished. The purpose of capture and detention is to remove from society and punish. The capital punishment issue could be resolved by placing all male capital criminals on one island and all female capital criminals on another island for the duration of their lives, to live a Robinson Crusoe existence without access to news of world activities. This would also be feasible for lesser crimes but for shorter terms. This would greatly reduce the cost of the penal system and remove from society the risk of escaped criminals and prison riots.

Mass Transit:

It is probably a mistake to concentrate efforts on transporting great masses into larger, more densely populated areas for their productive activities. We should not think only of now and only in terms of efficiency or the economics of association, but for the sake of future generations, give more consideration to human factors. The history of man demonstrates that he does not adjust well to crowding. Cities should be decentralized, spread out according to Federal standards. The next few decades should be spent limiting population centers by limiting the number of square feet of office space per city block and with such centers being no less than, say, 50 miles apart, probably arranged as squares or circles connected by high-speed rail systems. This should decrease traffic congestion, pollution and crime not to mention the favorable effect on mental health and domestic tranquility plus a degree of inherent defense from nuclear attack.

Nation's Capitol:

The nation is in need of a unifying project. It would be well to begin planning for a new Nation's Capitol to be constructed in a more central location. The present Capitol would become a museum center. Such a project would undoubtably touch the nation's fancy.

Government Academies:

The key to progress i.e. comfort and freedom is intelligence and wisdom. We have a complex, sophisticated, highly specialized society. Progress has produced specialists in all fields of endeavor and many of the more critical of the various specialties are licensed after demonstrating qualifications. But we delegate probably the most important task of all, government, to the untrained, the unlicensed. It's time to consider the establishment of "Democrat" and "Republican" Academies to be located in sites chosen by each party. Such academies would offer Ph.D degrees in Government. Such degrees would provide the Nation with men trained in Law, Economics, Diplomacy, Foreign Policy, Constitutional Law, Military Affairs and other areas in which they are called upon to exercise their office. Our present system does not give us such qualified Congressmen. These men must

be paid a salary commensurate with their training and responsibility. A degree from one of these academies would be a prerequisite for such offices as Congressman, Cabinet Member,
President, Supreme Court and possibly other high ranking offices.
Such men would be less susceptible to political pressure, and
more likely to respond to their intelligence and wisdom. It is
really no more logical to have untrained governing officials than
to have untrained persons practicing medicine or law.

The Vote:

Karl Marx made the statement that religion is the opiate of
the people. Presumably, he meant that religion keeps the people
sedate by providing a certain contentment with themselves and
their environment, a contentment which, according to his philosophy, is misleading as it prevents their striving for a "better
world of communism." The "Vote," by similar mechanism, works
to the contrary by lulling the people into believing that free
elections prevent communism. The vote is a wolf in sheep's
clothing. It provides a false sense of security, a feeling that it is
preserving freedom when, in fact, the reverse is true. The vote
is the mechanism by which democracies gradually deteriorate
into dictatorships. The majority exercise their liberty by voting,
but they vote for issues, for candidates, which favor tangible
material gain rather than the intangible freedom which they
already have. As noted in "The Vicious Circle," freedom is gradually eroded until, at some point, politics, through free elections
—the democratic process—produces a totalitarian government
which alone determines the national political ideology. The people, from that point, by their vote, determine, if anything, only
who will guide the country along that totalitarian course. This is
the reason Communists are so eager for all citizens to vote and
vote with ease, for all nations to become "democracies," a term
which they use very freely. If only the propertied, the responsible, the affluent vote, there is a much greater possibility that
liberty will be preserved because the affluent can "afford to consider and vote for the intangible freedom while the less respon-

sible, the "underprivileged," will vote away their freedom in favor of the tangible gain. They cannot "afford" to consider the luxury of the intangible freedom which they already have, anyway. Unfortunately, the affluent are outnumbered at the polls.

The United States has reached the point where the political course of the nation will not be altered by the presidential election process. The president could be elected by a toss of a coin insofar as the nation's political future is concerned. This is rapidly becoming true of Congress also. Free elections, the manifestation of the nation's desire to express its liberty, the means by which the individual has a voice in what rules and regulations he will live by, becomes the means by which he loses that voice. It makes no difference if the voter is eighteen, or even fifteen or fifty. The leftward swing did not start with the eighteen-year-old vote and will be only slightly accelerated by it. Franklin was wrong when he said, "We have given you a Republic, if *you* can keep it." The people will not keep a society free; free elections will not keep a society free. Only government, a government of highly qualified elected officials, who govern on the basis of knowledge, intelligence, and wisdom, rather than politics, can keep a nation free.

The hapless voters, the ones who really desire liberty, and desire to exercise that liberty by voting, over a few generations, vote themselves and their posterity into slavery.

The people therefore must be educated to the mechanics of the vicious circle so they will understand how to preserve their freedom.

These comments and proposals help to give a little more insight into the "socialization" process and to answer the three basic questions asked previously.

America is the only nation that can stop the motion of the vicious circle, a motion which gradually leads to totalitarianism. If American physicians will act to prevent socialized medicine, if conservatives will take the courses of action outlined above, then we might live to see falling arches of socialism all over the world as numerous Americans throw wrenches into the vicious circle.